Health Equality and
Social Justice in Old Age

of related interest

The Patient Revolution
How We Can Heal the Healthcare System
David Gilbert
ISBN 978 1 78592 538 2
eISBN 978 1 78450 932 3

Pain is Really Strange
Steve Haines
Illustrated by Sophie Standing
ISBN 978 1 84819 264 5
eISBN 978 0 85701 212 8

Positive Communication
Activities to Reduce Isolation and Improve Wellbeing of Older Adults
Robin Dynes
ISBN 978 1 78592 181 0
eISBN 978 1 78450 449 6

Dementia-Friendly Communities
Why We Need Them and How We Can Create Them
Susan H. McFadden, PhD
ISBN 978 1 78592 816 1
eISBN 978 1 78592 878 9

Person-Centred Thinking with Older People
Six Essential Practices
Helen Sanderson, Helen Bown and Gill Bailey
ISBN 978 1 84905 612 0
eISBN 978 1 78450 082 5

Supporting Older People Using Attachment-Informed and Strengths-Based Approaches
Imogen Blood and Lydia Guthrie
ISBN 978 1 78592 123 0
eISBN 978 1 78450 387 1

HEALTH EQUALITY and SOCIAL JUSTICE in OLD AGE

A FRONTLINE PERSPECTIVE

Dr Riaz Dharamshi

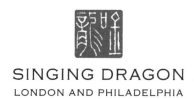

SINGING DRAGON
LONDON AND PHILADELPHIA

First published in Great Britain in 2023 by Singing Dragon,
an imprint of Jessica Kingsley Publishers
An Hachette Company

1

Copyright © Dr Riaz Dharamshi 2023

The right of Dr Riaz Dharamshi to be identified as the
Author of the Work has been asserted by him in accordance
with the Copyright, Designs and Patents Act 1988.

Front cover image source: Shutterstock®.

A CIP catalogue record for this title is available from the
British Library and the Library of Congress

ISBN 978 1 83997 365 9
eISBN 978 1 83997 381 9

Printed and bound in Great Britain by CPI Group UK

Jessica Kingsley Publishers' policy is to use papers that are natural,
renewable and recyclable products and made from wood grown in
sustainable forests. The logging and manufacturing processes are expected
to conform to the environmental regulations of the country of origin.

Jessica Kingsley Publishers
Carmelite House
50 Victoria Embankment
London EC4Y 0DZ

www.singingdragon.com

Contents

Introduction

Understanding science and medicine can teach you a lot about old age, but we should always be mindful of hubris. A technical understanding of illness does not constitute an emotional understanding of experience and the two should never be confused. Thus, in the practice of medicine, it is important always to remember that our patients will tell us the most important information: what it is like to be them.

Medical knowledge is a tool. It can also be a barrier. It can help diagnose and treat any number of medical problems, but it can also distract you from what really matters.

Old age is not defined only by the medical problems we experience. It is, instead, a very human experience – of ambitions, memories, passions and hopes. At its most basic level, medicine is a tussle with pathology – it either wins or loses. Life, however, is much more nuanced than that: in between the medical practitioner and the illness is a patient, and whatever the outcome, life has meaning to the person in the middle.

Good practice is founded on knowledge and experience, but great doctors transcend the empirical and master the softer skills of communication, empathy and engagement. I used to say that good doctors are the ones who are comfortable with uncertainty. Armed with this maxim, I strode confidently into the lives of my patients and told them that I knew what to do.

There was no moment when I realised I was wrong. What uncertainty? Whose uncertainty? Instead, there was the creeping awareness that my knowledge meant nothing unless I synchronised the rhythms of my practice to the needs of the person I was supposed to be helping. As a 30-something doctor, armed with his learning, what did I yet know about the hopes of someone in their late 80s? Perhaps I was gestated in the dying embers of a paternalistic medical culture, which meant that I was late to the realisation that doctors are not always the best arbiters of what a good outcome looks like. In fact, they often miss the point entirely.

It took me a while to articulate the problem. There are many strands. I was drawn into geriatric medicine by the understanding that older people are often poorly served. I saw that their care was too often determined by the shape of services rather than the shape of their needs. I saw how they were denied appropriate intervention, neglected by families, abused even; how they struggled for care, or even to have their problems taken seriously. I remember my anger when a junior doctor said to me, 'Are you the Care of the Smelly Registrar?' My feedback to him was forthright.

Yet, if the context for my commitment was clear in my own mind, the manner of my support was not. I landed, by instinct, on a model of advocacy that treated my patients as weak and incapable – people who needed an enforcer. It was a while before I understood that for all my good intentions, I was enacting the bias about older people prevalent across society: by speaking on their behalf, I was complicit in their loss of voice; by confidently representing what I thought were their needs, I was drowning out their own description. Older people don't need me to represent them, they need me to let them represent themselves.

Framed in this way, the challenges start to become a little clearer. One starts to look at how the organisation of our services affects the ability of my patients (our oldest and frailest neighbours) to access care: from how they get to hospital, to the clinic environment or the number of different specialists involved. The picture that emerges suggests that we are trying to make it hard for them.

A range of factors impede the delivery of good care, including workload, education and training, clinical record systems, staffing and systems of care. Fundamentally, however, you can only deliver good care if you understand what good looks like for each patient.

Not everyone wants the same outcome. Older people want different things. Some want to be pain free, to breathe a little easier, to make it to their granddaughter's wedding; others want to remain at home, to not go to hospital, to be with their cats. Some want me to do everything I can to cure them, while others want to die soon.

Therefore, the first lesson is that success looks like whatever your patient describes it as; and in aiming for such variation, you need to work in a healthcare system that allows for it. Not all variation is bad. All patients should be able to expect the same level of care, but not all patients will need it. But while I am trying to persuade you that the individual experience is paramount, I also need to impress on you the importance of our systems and habits of care. No one should be denied care or treatment because they are old; care and treatment should be chosen because they are right for the person. Involving patients effectively in the decisions about the care and treatment they receive results in the right care – and the right care often involves less intervention.

As medicine becomes ever more technical, the potential gap between what patients know and what doctors know widens, creating the risk of ever more delegation of decision-making to the technical experts. To some extent this is inevitable, but technical expertise should not be a pretext for loss of patient autonomy. I may know what is possible and how it could be achieved, but they know what is important. Technical excellence is essential, but by itself it is not enough. We need individualisation as well.

Our ability to respond to patients' individual needs asks also that we delegate responsibility, autonomy and judgement to the healthcare professionals who deal with them. Too often the nature of care is constrained by the organisation of our system, which, in myriad ways, prevents staff doing what they know is necessary. This can be understood in terms of both the scale of healthcare delivery and the nature of service management. In our drive for efficiency, patients are treated as units of need and staff as units of activity. This approach can squeeze out humanity.

Healthcare is a big, impersonal machine, but meaning is found in personal narratives. Threads of meaning are found wherever you go in healthcare, but they are easily lost. Observing the impacts of our care on real people is informative. A pain score chart is useful but nothing like seeing a patient comfortable enough to engage in conversation with their son for the last time.

The challenges on our health service are fundamentally demographic: we have an ageing population. The need to adapt to this reality is pressing but we should not be distracted. It is possible to enact a healthcare system that better deals with older people in larger numbers, but it does not require us to ignore their individual biographies.

Instead, I argue that it is precisely by understanding our individual patients better, and creating a more circumscribed role for healthcare in the lives of older people, that we will find our way to the kind of health service our population needs.

Over the coming pages, I want to trace for you some of the strands between old age as experienced now, old age as it could be experienced in the future and the current and future shape of healthcare services needed for them. While that may raise the spectre of a confusing entanglement, please do not despair: I propose simplicity. While particular issues may be complex, even complicated, there is always a straight line back to the patient.

Patients are our lodestar, and they will guide us through the discourse. The stories I present to you are drawn from my experiences as a doctor but are altered to protect patients' identities. They are there to serve as a reminder of what it is all about and a compass to direct us. But enough of the preamble, let us meet Yvonne.

Yvonne

I have known Yvonne for a few years now. Each time I see her, I am surprised that she is still going. The first time I met her, I was fairly certain her time was limited.

I try never to predict the future; patients like Yvonne remind you why not.

Four years ago, Yvonne was already tiny and physically frail. She lived in an ancient cottage nestled in the countryside. It was a July afternoon and I sat with her and her husband in their conservatory, looking out over the grazing sheep in the fields beyond.

Her GP wanted me to find out why she was losing weight and decide what to do about it. She confessed to a dull pain as I palpated the lower, right-hand quadrant of her abdomen. A CT scan showed something, but the radiologist was not entirely sure what – either a collection of infection or, possibly, a tumour. Antibiotics might clear any infection, but she didn't want to consider anything more involved. She did, however, agree to another scan a month later, to see if the shadow had disappeared. It had. There was no cancer.

Thereafter, I kept an eye on her and occasionally visited her if she became unwell. Over the next few years, she seemed to have shrunk a little more each time I saw her. Later, her memory and cognition had started to fail. She had trouble remembering me or what we had discussed; she was disorientated in time and started to forget the names of friends and relatives. She remained anchored in reality by her husband and their cat, Monty.

A little while ago, I was doing a round in the local acute hospital, and I saw her. A tiny slip, lying in bed. She had the haunted, wind-swept look of someone with advanced dementia. Her husband told me that the doctors had seen her and decided, with his agreement, not to treat her infection and to let her die in comfort. It was a good plan, except for the fact that Yvonne didn't die. Without any treat-ment, she recovered and returned home.

She still seems to be shrinking, and I keep imagining that one day, perhaps soon, perhaps later, she will have become so small that she simply disappears, in a little puff.

CHAPTER I

Death

The moment of death is unmistakable. The uninitiated watch the breathing. The more familiar look at the face: life is visible in even the least animated human face – it is in the tone of the muscles and the spark of the eyes, and it is these that evaporate at the moment of extinction. There is something spiritual about witnessing death. A Cartesian would reference the exit of the soul from the body, and it takes a staunch materialist to think of dying only in terms of blood flow, enzymes and neurones. Life, and therefore death, is a function only of biology, but life as a human takes us a little beyond the simple mechanics of being: we imbue it with meaning, purpose, family and friends, and we elevate it through the simple expedient of our glorious language. Humans are storytellers, capable of infinite cognitive wonders. And as Ernest Becker[1] reminds us, we are forever grounded by being trapped in our mortal bodies. There is much ground to cover, but let us for now remain at the moment of death.

There is a profound intimacy to being present at the end of a life. It is a gossamer instant: utterly distinctive, entirely permanent, with the suggestion of the unreal. The transition from living to dead takes seconds and then immediately takes on the sheen of the unbelievable: it is unbelievable that the body in front of you was, moments before, a living being. A recently deceased person has all the elements of life but has lost the delicate synchrony that kept them chugging away.

Medical practice demands that I go through set motions to confirm that the dead person in front of me is dead: I am obliged to check for a pulse, breathing, pupillary reflexes and a response to physical stimulus. I have yet to find someone alive, but I have often appreciated those quiet seconds to think for a short while on the person that was. I often think of the road that led them to that point, to which I and my colleagues have borne witness.

I am a geriatrician; it is my great privilege to look after older people with frailty. We are perhaps an unfashionable bunch, because we intrinsically accept the limits of human ingenuity and medical technology to forestall the ravages of time. We are the people who ask, 'Who is the person to whom this is happening?' rather than just, 'What is the medical problem?' For it is only by understanding the needs and wants of the older person in front of you that you can hope to understand how to apply the science of medicine. I call it science, but in practice it feels more like art – we geriatricians have our idiosyncrasies and, for all the empiricism with which we are imbued throughout medical training, we often practise in an evidence-free zone: no one has really explored the impact of our treatments on our patients, with their advanced age and multiple and complex problems. We extrapolate the evidence base from the younger, single-pathology trial groups, or we have no evidence to refer to at all.

The burning point is that senescence and frailty change everything in medicine. One may consider a pneumonia to be simply a chest infection, whomever it happens to, but pneumonia in someone frail is a great deal more than that. A failing body is both more susceptible to infections and less capable of fighting them. A failing body is less responsive to medical treatment and more prone to complications. A few years ago, before COVID-19, a succession of my patients contracted a strain of influenza against which they had been inoculated. They mounted none of the immune response to the vaccine that I did. So, while they serially succumbed, I sailed through the clouds of infected secretions flying out of their lungs unscathed. The coronavirus pandemic has taught us all a little more respect for infections against which we have little immune protection.

Those of you who work with older people will hopefully recognise my point of view; the challenge for all of us is how we counter clinical nihilism. Based only on first appearances, it would be easy to discount the prospect of recovery in any of our patients. The skill of caring for those with frailty is understanding when to fight and when to fold. We are, of course, guided by evidence, and for all my glibness, geriatrics is underpinned by established and effective modes of practice. But I am not writing a textbook on geriatrics. I want us to dive into the philosophy and phenomenology of ageing to inform our practice. I want to learn from the experiences of my patients and their relatives and to channel the lessons from them into my own understanding of how we care for older people. One's approach to a patient is informed by a great deal more than just the medicine – one must account for the goals of the person, their risk-taking style, their philosophy even. For there is rarely a right answer – there is only the answer that best approximates the patient's version of perfect.

Let me tell you about May. May was a 95-year-old lady, whom I had last seen six months before, when she had recovered poorly from a hip fracture. She had reluctantly agreed to move out of her flat into a nursing home. It was not what she wanted, and it was not what I wanted, but we live in an imperfect world. She had been a drama teacher in her younger days, and even through the parched, papery skin and wasted muscles, one could see that she had been an elegant and attractive woman. For all her physical frailty, she was intellectually terrifying, and she would verbally spar with me on my ward rounds as a means of distracting me from doing any medicine on her: she was afraid I would only mess things up for her by trying to get her better.

Since her discharge from my care, she had lived in suspended animation in her new nursing home, where she bore the indignity of being surrounded by ailing elders phlegmatically. It came as something of a relief to her when she contracted pneumonia. She thought that it was her chance to exit gracefully.

I don't believe in fate, but the evidence for Sod's Law is sometimes compelling. I think May would agree with me: the care home staff would not leave her to die and called an ambulance. The ambulance crew, having been summoned, and finding a very poorly lady, did what they often do and whisked her off to hospital. I can imagine her plaintive cries being ignored all the way.

It is the fashion in Emergency Departments (EDs) these days to treat with haste, but it is to May's eternal credit that she found the strength to be noticed. I can imagine the agitation among the ED staff to take blood samples, send her off to X-ray and start antibiotics. She received none of these things: she refused and requested politely but unshakeably to be sent back to her home, where she could get on with dying in her own way.

It is common for older people to be denied their autonomy when the mechanism of the acute medical response kicks in, and there was a great deal of chin scratching about this feisty old lady who would not let the doctors do what doctors do. They questioned her capacity to decide, they checked she understood that she had a treatable medical problem and they required her to use her limited reserves to resist their advances.

The ED doctors eventually relented. But Sod was not done with her yet: her nursing home refused to have her back. They said they could not meet her needs. That is how we came to meet – when she was transferred to a community hospital in which I worked. And still Sod had more to give: while waiting for an ambulance to bring her to my hospital, one of the staff saw her coughing after taking a drink, and she was placed nil by mouth to reduce her risk of aspirating fluid into her lungs. Bad decisions in healthcare result from ignorance, scarcity of time and risk aversion. All three were in play with that particular action. Who in their right mind would deny a dying woman a drink of water?

When I saw her the next day, she was annoyed: annoyed at not being allowed home, annoyed at not being allowed to drink and annoyed that she was still alive.

I chatted with her and agreed that she need not have treatment, that she could have fluids, which we would help her take as safely as possible, and that she was welcome to die under our care any time she liked. She was easy to talk to about death – she was a forthright woman.

May was bright and talented and told rip-roaring stories of her past. She was unafraid of death, but most importantly, she was ready. We spoke about family visits while she was in hospital, and she was quite happy for her daughter to spend as much time with her as she wanted but did not want her grandchildren to see her. She wanted them to remember her the way she used to be, not as a fading body in a hospital gown with a woolly hat on. I accused her, jokingly, of vanity, and she told me to sod off. She died peacefully three days later.

May is a case study in good intentions with bad implementation. Before she had moved into the care home, we had spent time with her outlining what we would and wouldn't do for her should she become poorly again. We had agreed that whatever happened to her, we would support her to stay in her care home. Yet when she became sick, the staff were worried about looking after her. We succeeded in allowing her to die, but not before putting her part way through the medical machine. She did well not to be chewed up by it.

Modern medicine exists to diagnose and cure. We have changed the shape and nature of many illnesses, but we have not cheated death. Major developments in sanitation, education, employment and public health have transformed the shape of our society:[2] in Dorset, 29% of the population is over the age of 65, compared with 5% under the age of five.[3] The figures tell us something about the prevalence of age in our society, but the story is not in the headlines, it is in the biography of real lives and real deaths.

Modern medicine has appropriated death. Perhaps, amid the

medico-technological revolutions of the 20th Century, we have bought into the idea that death can be forestalled in hospital. Today, almost half of deaths take place in hospitals from illnesses such as heart disease, stroke and dementia.[4] A fifth of deaths take place in care homes and 6% in hospices, while only a quarter of people die in their own homes.[5] A hundred years ago, two-thirds of deaths were caused by infectious diseases, and the majority died at home.[6] We die in hospitals not because we choose to, but because hospitals are where people go when they are ill.

It is in hospitals that death has become shrouded, invisible even. Sherwin Nuland[7] argues that medicine has altered our thinking about death. Shielded by victories over infant mortality and infectious illnesses, medicine has created the narrative of our fight against illness and disease, giving lie to the fundamental truth that death can be delayed but it cannot be prevented. Our medical practice is represented by a figurative battle with death rather than an honest parley with it.

The primary mistake is to consider the aged person as a collection of discrete illnesses. The clumsy watchword in geriatrics is 'multi-morbidity', which references the reality that as people age, they accumulate medical problems. A patient of mine will commonly have a mixture of hypertension, diabetes, dementia, ischaemic heart disease, renal impairment, osteoporosis, atrial fibrillation and so on. Each disease has its own set of guidelines to follow, which invariably results in numerous medications, many of which will counteract the effects of the others. A classic example is the frail patient on multiple blood pressure medications, which then increase the risk of low blood pressure, which causes falls. A fall in someone with osteoporosis can lead to a fractured hip, whereas you or I would sustain mild bruising. In older patients with a hip fracture, 10% will be dead within a month and 30% within a year.[8]

To treat multiple, separate pathologies in a single person individually is to recklessly miss the point. I joke sometimes that I spend 50%

of my time reversing medical complications and 50% stopping new ones. Multimorbidity viewed from sufficient altitude is indicative of the failure of a complex system. In his book, *Being Mortal*, Atul Gawande quotes Leonid Gavrilov, who argues that humans fail the way all complex systems fail: 'gradually and randomly'.[9]

Frailty and multimorbidity are the gradual and random failure of a complex system. Understanding senescence in this way can have a profound impact on the way one practises medicine. Rather than viewing each new illness, disease or complication as a brand-new fight, each one is an additional biological detail in a complex whole. Boiled down to its reductive end point, effectively managing the failure of my patient's complex system starts with the simple question, 'What does success look like for this person?'

May tried to make the asking of the question redundant, but in the matrix of single-pathology focus, and the efficient and relentless momentum of the emergency response, her quiet but steady voice was not heard at all clearly. May is an exemplar of the need for modern medics to be honest about the limits of medical efficacy. We did not need to be honest with her, we needed to be honest with ourselves.

However, I cannot shake the impression that we are recasting ourselves as a technological species; as people like George Monbiot[10] outline the impact of our collective behaviours on climate and species destruction, I am struck by the tacit assumption aired in conversation that cure lies not in our behaviours and choices but in having the patience to wait for technological solutions. It is the same outsourcing of agency that comes into play in the role of medical services in managing the process of dying and death. We have entrusted the expertise of managing illness in all its forms to our technological model of medical practice, while giving too little thought to the softer, social elements involved in managing mortality. It is a covenant that belies elements of our fundamental nature.

In *Sapiens: A Brief History of Humankind*,[11] Yuval Harari argues that humans are distinguished not simply by their ability to think in the abstract and communicate in infinite possible ways through language, but also by their ability to use these skills to collaborate across distance and numbers. He proposes our capacity to share stories as the mechanism through which we do this. It is our ability to orchestrate in large groups towards a shared goal that defines us, through the subscription of shared goals. Ever since communities began, we have belonged to shared religions, mythologies and social movements. What is it that unites us today? Individualism? Capitalism? Mammon? It rather depends on your optimism about the human condition.

In the trailer to his radio series, *A History of the World in 100 Objects*,[12] Neil MacGregor emblematically remarked that, 'Ever since humans have been making objects, they have been making beautiful objects.' Think of cave art and how the blown handprints seem to reach across aeons with tenderness. I offer this as a counterpoint to the projection of humans as a technological species in an arms race against illness and ageing. One cannot discount the human capacity for ingenuity, but should one really rely on it? The history of human civilisation is not one of relentless progress but of cyclical waxing and waning. One wonders if we are prepared for the possibility of the waning of our individual selves after our recent burst of collective progress.

May was prepared, but some of the people who served her in her final illness were not, and it was May who bore the brunt of our systemic intransigence.

May's challenge to us is to navigate our path towards technical excellence in conjunction with the sensitive acknowledgement of futility and recognition that one's definition of success is altered by one's personal perspective. Quantity of life may be trumped by quality of life, and even quality of death, and knowing when this is the case comes from the simplest of places. We need to create the time and awareness to ask of all our patients, 'What really matters to you?'

Endnotes

1 Becker, E. (1973) *The Denial of Death*. London: Souvenir Press.

2 Raleigh, V. (2021) *What is Happening to Life Expectancy in England?* London: The King's Fund. Accessed on 7/3/2022 at www.kingsfund.org.uk/publications/ whats-happening-life-expectancy-england.

3 Dorset County Council (2018) *Our Communities Topic Report: 2017 Mid-Year Population Estimates in Dorset*. Accessed on 7/2/2022 at https://apps.geowessex. com/stats/Reports/Topic/Older-People.

4 Public Health England (2017) 'Major Causes of Death and How They Have Changed.' In *Health Profile for England: 2017* (Chapter 2). Accessed on 7/2/2022 at www.gov.uk/government/publications/health-profile-for-england/chapter-2-major-causes-of-death-and-how-they-have-changed#trends-in-leading-causes-of-death.

5 Public Health England (2018) *Statistical Commentary: End of Life Care Profiles, February 2018 Update*. Accessed on 7/2/2022 at www.gov.uk/government/ statistics/end-of-life-care-profiles-february-2018-update.

6 Baillie, L. and Howe, E. (2012) *Causes of Death: A Study of a Century of Change in England and Wales*. Office of Health Economics. Accessed on 7/2/2022 at www. ohe.org/publications/causes-death-study-century-change-england-and-wales.

7 Nuland, S. B. (1994) *How We Die*. London: Vintage.

8 Lisk, R. and Yeong, K. (2014) 'Reducing mortality from hip fracture: A systematic quality improvement programme.' *BMJ Quality Improvement 3*, u205006.w2103.

9 Gawande, A. (2014) *Being Mortal: Illness, Medicine and What Matters in the End*. London: Profile Books, p.33.

10 Monbiot, G. (2018) *Out of the Wreckage*. New York: Verso Books.

11 Harari, Y. (2015) *Sapiens: A Brief History of Humankind*. New York: Harper.

12 BBC (2010) *A History of the World in 100 Objects*. BBC Radio 4. Accessed on 7/2/2022 at www.bbc.co.uk/programmes/b00nrtd2.

Arthur and Mildred

When I met Arthur, he was 92. His wife, Mildred, was 87 yet suffered with worse health. They had aged together in a bungalow in Bridport. Over the course of 60 years, the paraphernalia of life had accumulated – most of it dated and out of place in the 21st Century: heavy mahogany furniture that seemed to suck the light out of the room, looming over the space. Arthur and Mildred were from a generation that still considered eating to be an activity requiring its own space and scheduling: dining took place in a dining room, undistracted from other activities. Their dining table was large enough to seat eight, yet it rarely did. It was now piled high with papers, signalling their loss in the fight to stay ahead of the tidal wave of detritus that swamps modern life.

As a result, in their waning years of tottering mobility, they continued to live in a home overrun with furniture they neither used nor needed and found the weeds of bills, paperwork and junk mail sprouting around them. Only a single track between the kitchen and living room was unblighted by furniture and only a single area of floor between their easy chairs and the television was visible to the naked eye, revealing a high quality but highly aged beige Axminster carpet.

The day-to-day experience of life for both Arthur and Mildred was challenged by more than just their physical clutter – were it not for the ravages of time on their bodies, they might have navigated the house easily. Yet their desire to tame their surroundings was scuppered by the realities of old age. Arthur was a retired engineer, who used to stand at 6 ft. 2 but was now stooped in a question-mark shape short of 5 ft. 9. He was riddled with arthritis, which left his hands gnarled, his back and hips creaking and his knees with the tendency to give way underneath him. In spite of his relative loss of height, the stiffness in his limbs and joints meant that although he could see the physical continuity between his lower legs and the rest of his body, his inability to reach them meant that, to him, they were only philosophically part of him. With the equipment given to him by the occupational therapist, he was able to get by. The leg lifter, long shoehorn and sock tool were the lifesavers he never thought he would need. Who knew that one could reach a point in life when donning socks independently would be a triumph?

Arthur would never admit it, but it was looking after his wife that caused him the most anxiety. Their 62 years of marriage meant that he could never contemplate life without her. He would certainly miss her terribly if she were gone, but there would be benefits too. Mildred's memory was not what it used to be, but that did not stop them reminiscing about the past. Indeed, there was a great deal to remember fondly.

They were a couple who had experienced great contentment and fun together. Arthur's job had taken them, for a while, all over the world in his senior position at a petrochemical company. Their children had thrived and succeeded and gave them immense pride. But in the present, Mildred was less reliable. Arthur could cope with her memory lapses, but her physical limitations tested him more.

The second half of Mildred's life had been if not defined then certainly influenced by her type 2 diabetes. The management of one's blood sugars is only half the challenge of living with the condition in old age. The other half is dealing with the effects on the body of the long-term diabetes. Mildred in particular had been affected by poor eyesight from diabetic retinopathy, but more profound than even her partial blindness was the autonomic dysfunction, which meant that her body became less able to maintain a stable blood pressure when she changed posture. Thus, when she stood up, her blood pressure would often fall catastrophically, causing her to collapse. The lack of blood supply to her brain could be transiently significant, leading to loss of consciousness and even fitting.

Over the last few years, Arthur had learned to recognise these events and, rather than seeking medical help, would put a cushion under her head until she came round a few moments later and then gently help her back to her feet when she had recovered enough to give it a try. Latterly, however, Mildred had become unable to get up without help, and he had become unable to help her himself. He reasoned that there was little sense in them both ending up in a pile on the floor.

The week before I met the couple, Mildred had collapsed. Unfazed by this now familiar event, Arthur had considered his options. With Mildred lying with her head on the hearth, Arthur concluded too high a degree of hazard to help her up again. As many of us in his situation would, Arthur called 999, hoping to request the assistance of a paramedic to help him return Mildred to the upright position.

However, he reckoned without the unthinking application of the ambulance service's algorithm. Asked whether he could feel Mildred's pulse, Arthur demurred. In the heat of an urgency that existed only in the logic of a computer program inadequately supervised by a thinking human, the call handler did not stop to enquire why Arthur could not feel a pulse (he could not bend down) and shouted at Arthur to start cardiopulmonary resuscitation (CPR).

Raised as he was to show good manners in all situations, Arthur did not correct the mistake and did as he was told. Creaking himself down to his knees, he began chest compressions on a woman he knew to have fainted, because a call handler who could not see what was actually occurring knew she had suffered a cardiac arrest.

By this time, matters had been taken out of Arthur's hands: within minutes, his house had been breached by a paramedic from a rapid response ambulance car, an ambulance crew arriving separately and two policemen who had been cruising nearby in their patrol car.

For 45 minutes, they checked his wife over, before telling him that she had fainted.

'I appreciated their help, doctor,' he told me a week later, 'but it does seem like an awful waste of resources. Can you tell me how I might get someone over in future to help me pick her up without starting World War 3?'

This is the lot of people like Arthur.

CHAPTER 2

The Invention of Old Age

We are infants in the business of ageing. We are taking our first tottering steps towards understanding the mechanics of longevity. We have always had old people but never of the volume and vintage that we have today. Most improvements in human life expectancy have been achieved in the last 125 years, covering only five generations.[1] The human species is about 8000 generations old. We are still discovering the practicalities of our new durability and are a long way off mastering them.

Since the mid-1800s, the rate of progress in life expectancy has been linear,[2] to the extent that we are less similar now to our forebears, in terms of mortality profiles, than they were to chimpanzees.[3] It is not us that has changed, it is our environments. Five generations are too few to enact genetic change. Our prehistoric ancestors may well recognise us, but would they recognise the habitats we have created?

Older people used to be a rare commodity, relied upon as sources of wisdom and tradition.[4] They have always been there, but it is only now that one wonders if there should be a collective noun for them. In 1917, George V sent 24 telegrams to subjects reaching the age of 100;[5] in 2017, Elizabeth II sent out 14,910,[6] so it is little wonder that the Department for Work and Pensions has a dedicated 'Centenarian Team'.[7]

We are therefore inexperienced practitioners in the business of being old, and senescence is not really part of our biography. Until recently, we were a species whose individuals burned brightly but more briefly, with occasional aged outliers. The very old have always existed but not in the numbers we see today. How we adapt to communities a quarter constructed of older people is wisdom we must acquire de novo. This novelty may ignite pangs of optimism – that ageing and frailty are simply fresh medical problems in search of solutions.

It is a statement that lacks face validity, but one cannot prove the negative. One can only start with what is currently known about ageing. The remarkable rise in the endurance of individual human lives speaks to the plasticity of human mortality in response to significant environmental changes. Yet no humans live without ageing. The gradual wearing away of physical condition reduces us at varying rates to the enfeebled state of advanced old age. The most popular models of frailty in humans refer to cumulative deficits[8] and the phenotype of ageing.[9] Both are descriptive rather than explanatory and attempt to describe in detail what is easy to see in outline.

The ubiquity of ageing across multicellular species creates the impression of purpose – but we must be wary of divining purpose in natural selection. Its characterisation as a 'blind watchmaker'[10] remains apt. Natural selection is without meaning. It is simply the emergent mechanism for the propagation and perpetuation of living organisms. The beautiful variety of nature (the sentiment is mine) enlists any tool that improves survival and reproduction in a world with competition for resources. Yet virtually no multicellular organism has leveraged immortality.

Leonid Gavrilov[11] suggests that ageing can be considered primarily as a function of evolution, with the precise processes by which it is enacted being of secondary importance. Thus, ageing should be viewed from the perspective of evolutionary imperative rather than degradation of telomeres or mitochondrial decay, for example.

In this barely sufficient primer of the evolution of ageing, it is Medawar's Mutation Accumulation Theory[12] and Williams' later Antagonistic Pleiotropy Theory[13] that are our starting points. The former asserts that deleterious genes that act in infancy, prior to reproductive age, will be selected against, while adverse gene mutations that only surface in later life, after the main period of reproductive activity, will not be weeded out due to their manifestation after offspring have emerged. The tendency for late-acting genes to be overlooked by natural selection will lead to the gradual accumulation of deleterious genes surfacing in old age, giving rise to the phenotype of ageing. Antagonistic Pleiotropy Theory extends this initial idea by suggesting that detrimental, late-acting genes confer a selective advantage in early life and are therefore positively selected for.

It seems dangerous to explain a past we can never know, and the acceptance of an evolutionary theory of ageing will depend to some extent on your benevolence to evolutionary explanations. Consider, in the context of near-universal mortality, the possible mechanisms that could explain senescence and death. Consider also that the majority of animals in the wild do not die of old age but disease, predation or mishap. If animals were programmed to die at a set time, the risk of death would rise precipitously above a certain age. We do not see this in humans, and we do not see it in animals in captivity, which tend to live longer than their wild counterparts. Death rates in old age are not greatly increased – the annual risk of death for a Japanese 65-year-old is 0.8%.[14]

Ronald Lee[15] has extended the idea of the evolution of ageing from these classic theories by arguing that post-reproductive survival is selected for, through the investment in children by parents, grandparents and social groups: he asserts that the intergenerational transfer of resources increases the individual chances of survival to reproductive maturity. If one imagines that a child is more likely to survive with the support of an extended family or social group, one can begin to imagine how post-reproductive survival becomes evolutionarily important. Lee offers us little on the process of ageing but shows us one interpretation of the function, over millennia, of older people in the success of social groups.

It is this theoretical position that overlays with my lived experience. There seems to be an imperative to ageing that has to be seen in the right context to be understood. Viewed by themselves, older people are people no longer capable of doing what they used to do. Increasingly, modern society hives off its older people to live alone at home, in retirement villages or in care homes. Their wider role has been degraded over time so that they are, increasingly, shadow operatives in the daily community life. Juxtapose this rough sketch of contemporary life for the older people with their reaction to children.

A few years ago, I took my two-year-old daughter into work with me, where the staff and patients made an appropriate fuss of her. She ran up and down the corridors and was fascinated by the fish tank. With the patient's permission, she saw me examine someone's abdomen, and later told the nursery school staff that, 'Daddy is a doctor; he dusts patients' tummies.' More remarkable, however, was the effect she had on the patients. People with advanced dementia, who could not remember me week to week, would ask me how Eliza was the next time I saw them. One lady spent a week furiously knitting a Samuel Whiskers teddy (Eliza prefers the more villainous Beatrix Potter characters) to have it ready for my next ward round.

More recently, one of the ward healthcare assistants would bring her gorgeous baby into work, and I would take him off her, tuck him under my arm and continue my ward round. The effect he had on the patients was transformative. Some smiled, some cried, but he lit up the ward and animated their days. Theirs was joy without affect. The pop psychologist in me tends towards explanations about regeneration and renewal, but we needn't resort to fanciful, emotive explanations. It may be understood purely in terms of the evolution of social function: Lee's theory suggests that prosperous populations will tend to select for individuals who contribute to the success of the group, resulting in communities in which older people are invested in the ascendancy of children – indeed, they are programmed for it.

However, it seems churlish to dismiss older people's joy in the face of babies and toddlers in terms only of biology. The satisfaction of continuation acts as a counterpoint to the reality of their own impending demise.

I recall Graham, a gregarious gentleman, knocked horizontal by one of the most brutal manifestations of a stroke. Strokes have a predilection for our language centres. With our broad-brush characterisation of brain function, we distinguish between the areas of the brain responsible for the understanding of language and the areas of the brain responsible for the production of language, including the coordination of the muscles of speech. This is called dysphasia, and I have yet to determine whether receptive dysphasia (the inability to understand language) or expressive dysphasia (the inability to communicate with speech) is worse. One lady I met had a total aphasia and yet seemed perfectly content to sit there knitting. So fluent was her knitting that I am sure I could divine meaning and sentiment through the manner of movement of her knitting needles: her normally languid needle strokes would occasionally hit a peak of fervour or energy when she was bothered by something.

Graham, however, had expressive dysphasia – he could understand almost everything you said but struggled to articulate anything of note. By sheer force of personality, he would expel words that indicated what he was trying to say. The complexities of the circuitry of the brain are best revealed when it malfunctions. Graham, for example, referred to 'The Duchess' instead of 'my wife'. I would repeat back to him what he had said and hearing me repeat his semantic misplacements would make him smile.

On one of the ward rounds with the baby under my arm, Graham was moved to tears. The baby was quite content to hold Graham's hand for a few moments. All Graham could say was, 'It's OK now.' He died a week later.

Elisabeth Kübler-Ross[16] states that in our unconscious minds we cannot die, we can only be killed. We heighten the impact of our instinctive denial through modern, western, social norms in which death is unacknowledged and children are shielded from the universal truth of mortality. We recast death in the language of the reversible (she's gone to a better place), thus revealing a contemporary failure to accept life as finite.

However, we should not despair. Patients like Graham indicate that it is possible to confront death and accept it. Indeed, time spent in the grip of advanced frailty requires people to face up to their impermanence. Kübler-Ross sheds light on this phenomenon through her description of the dying role: as people face death, they want to pass on stories, share wisdom and make peace.[17] Linda Emanuel and Karen Scandrett[18] take us a little further by reminding us that modern medicine has forgotten about the dying role and that by medicalising death, we rob our patients of the opportunity to run through the important steps towards a peaceful death. Graham made peace, but not through my design – the opportune visit of a cute little boy provided the substrate for him to decide that the future of the world lay before children like the one he saw that day.

Patients die differently, and Graham is perhaps unusual. However, he indicates to us what is possible. He was not typically ready to die – he had not consistently expressed his own readiness to die over time. Yet, he moved himself into the dying role and died peacefully; I think he was content at the end. Some of this was achieved by chance but even then, we still deserve a little credit: how often are the efforts of older patients to navigate through the dying role undermined by the well-intentioned but poorly reasoned efforts of the healthcare system and their families to save their lives?

It becomes our professional and social duty to recognise futility and invest in appropriate care at any stage of life. For the frail, there comes a point at which we need to accept reality and value dignity and comfort over defiance and heroics. The state of the art in geriatrics revolves less around the reversal of ageing and more around its accommodation. Frailty is largely unmalleable with the tools of modern medicine; we could, however, be very good at supporting patients to live with their frailty and optimise medical input around the factors that can be modified. At the same time, we can recognise that each of us has limited time and the needs of the individual should not be subsumed by the imperative of a health system that has evolved to attempt cure at any cost. This is not to advocate for perpetual negativity in the care of the seniors: David Oliver[19] recalled treating a patient who reported to him that he was 'considerably transformed' following treatment for an acute medical problem. Instead, the element of surprise and chance in the outcome for older people is mitigated by a system that follows people over time so that their presentation with sudden illness is framed by an understanding of what they are like when they are well. It is biographical information of this type that underpins good decision-making in the care of older people and transforms practice from one founded on inaccurate assumptions based on age to accurate assessments predicated on individual knowledge.

Endnotes

1 Burger, O., Baudisch, A. and Vaupel, J. W. (2012) 'Human mortality improvement in evolutionary context.' *Proceedings of the National Academy of Sciences of the United States of America 109*, 44, 18210–18214.

2 Oeppen, J. and Vaupel, J. W. (2002) 'Demography: Broken limits to life expectancy.' *Science 296*, 1029–1031.

3 Burger, Baudisch and Vaupel (2012).

4 Warraich, H. (2017) *Modern Death: How Medicine Changed the End of Life.* New York: St Martin's Press.

5 Royal Statistical Society (2013) *How Many Telegrams, Maam?* Accessed on 13/2/2019 at www.statslife.org.uk/features/54-how-many-telegrams-maam.

6 Siddique, H. (2017) 'Centenarians are fastest growing age group in UK, figures show.' *The Guardian*. Accessed on 7/2/2022 at www.theguardian.com/society/2017/sep/27/rise-in-uk-life-expectancy-slows-significantly-figures-show.

7   Bingham, J. (2014) 'Queen's "birthday care team" expands to cope with surge of 100 years olds.' *The Telegraph*. Accessed on 7/2/2022 at www.telegraph.co.uk/news/health/elder/11121184/Queens-birthday-card-team-expands-to-cope-with-surge-of-100-year-olds.html.

8   Rockwood, K. and Mitnitski, A. (2007) 'Frailty in relation to the accumulation of deficits.' *The Journals of Gerontology, Series A 62*, 7, 722–727.

9   Fried, L. P., Tangen, C. M., Walston, J., Newman, A. B. *et al.* (2001) 'Frailty in older adults: Evidence for a phenotype.' *The Journals of Gerontology, Series A 56*, 3, M146–M157.

10   Dawkins, R. (1986) *The Blind Watchmaker*. New York: Norton.

11   Gavrilov, L. A. and Gavrilova, N. S. (2002) 'Evolutionary theories of aging and longevity.' *The Scientific World Journal 2*, 339–356.

12   Medawar, P. B. (1946) 'Old age and natural death.' *Modern Q 1*, 30–56.

13   Williams, G. C. (1957) 'Pleiotropy, natural selection and the evolution of senescence.' *Evolution 11*, 398–411.

14   Burger, Baudisch and Vaupel (2012).

15   Lee, R. (2003) 'Rethinking the evolutionary theory of aging: Transfers, not births, shape senescence in social species.' *Proceedings of the National Academy of Sciences of the United States of America 100*, 16, 9637–9642.

16   Kübler-Ross, E. (1969) *On Death and Dying*. New York: The MacMillan Company.

17   *Ibid.*

18   Emanuel, L. and Scandrett, K. G. (2010) 'Decisions at the end of life: Have we come of age?' *BMC Medicine 8*, 57.

19   Oliver, D. (2020) '"Considerably transformed" – changing the narrative on admitting older patients.' *British Medical Journal 368*, m652.

Ronald

Ronald was a faller and a fairly spectacular one at that. The first time he fell, he broke his pelvis into two pieces. The second time, he shattered it – there was little point in counting the pieces. A cursory glance at the X-ray revealed that it was all a bit of a mess. The third time, his iliac crest (the large wing of bone at the back of the pelvis) was split into two, like a coconut.

The management of pelvic fractures, even ones as comprehensive as Ronald's, is simple: control their pain, pre-emptively manage constipation and get them on their feet. Empathise, sympathise, cajole and occasionally bark. Do whatever works to get them out of bed and walking. Bed rest is a one-way route to muscle wastage, deconditioning and permanent immobility.

Indolence, however, was not Ronald's problem. Indeed, over the course of a year, he subjected his skeleton to serial battery. If anything, he was too mobile. We had made a number of suggestions to help him walk more safely – from using a Zimmer frame to having a riser-recliner chair to make standing up less hazardous, plus a number of adaptations to his bathroom to make the process of washing and dressing safer: on one occasion, he had fallen in his bathroom and then sustained a mild head injury when the friend who found him opened the bathroom door on his head. Even Ronald could laugh about that one.

Yet, Ronald was steadfast. He thanked us for our help and advice but declined all of the adaptations we suggested. The right of the frailest and oldest members of our communities to choose the interventions they accept from us is a hill worth defending. Too often the rights and autonomy of older people and those with frailty are buried underneath the overwhelming insistence of family and healthcare professionals, all in the name of 'managing risk'. But whose risk is it?

Better still is to understand the context for the decisions being made. A hospital bed on a ward is my home turf. It disempowers patients. I therefore asked Ronald if I could follow him up at home to see how he was getting on. He readily agreed.

I love seeing patients at home. They are more relaxed – after all, in their own homes, they are in charge. As soon as I walk in, I can tell how well they are managing day-to-day life. I tend, also, to get a better sense from them about the problems that need addressing.

A week or two later, as I drove up to Ronald's house, I knew immediately the source of Ronald's steadfastness. It was a beautiful home. The driveway curved in a circle around a central island of brightly coloured flowers. It was a 1930s Art Deco house, and while the shell of the house was rather simple, the details – they were spectacular. The door knocker was a Mackintosh moustache motif, and the floor was a deep, polished parquet. You could sense the depth of the wooden blocks under your feet – I wanted to bend down and touch them. Paintings were everywhere. One often sees paintings in the homes of patients – usually their own. The quality varies, and there tends to be a limited range of subject matter: landscapes, animals and still life. But here, in Ronald's house, was a wonderful variety of abstracts, historical pieces and portraits from a bunch of different artists. I didn't recognise any in particular, but the whiff of quality was apparent. Even with no technical training, one can distinguish the 'good' art from the 'bad'.

Ronald was sat in his easy chair obliquely in front of the large stone fireplace, which dwarfed his television. The fire surround was another Mackintosh motif. Scattered around the large, light sitting room was a collection of pots and vases – some with intricate painted designs, others with wonderful glazed patinas. Ronald was bathed in the light that flooded through the large French windows that opened on to a three-terraced lawn, manicured and precise, bordered by well-tended flower beds. My granny was a botanist, and she would have thrilled at the plants on show. All I know is that they looked lovely.

It was more than a wonderful home: it was his late wife's magnum opus. She had been an interior designer, and this house, or at least its interior and gardens, were her present to him when he retired. It was both a charming place to live and a memento of her. By remaining in the house, Ronald felt closer to his wife, whom he still missed terribly.

It was immediately clear why he would not allow the adaptations we had recommended: he did not want the balance and precision of his wife's legacy to be ruined. It had already been a big step for him to accept the chair that rather jarred with the overall feel of the room. That was a concession he had been loath to make.

For some older people, like Ronald, the acceptance of help is a statement of defeat. It is, to them, the first step on a pathway that leads, inevitably, to living in a care home. They worry that by allowing services into their homes, they leave the door ajar for health and social services to wear away at them, to coerce or crowbar them out of their homes and into a nursing home.

Defiance gets them a long way, but perhaps not far enough. There comes a point where subsistence independently becomes impossible. Ronald wanted to continue as he had done since his wife died. He wanted to remain in the place where he felt most connected to her. To take him away from her would be the end of meaning for him, and he did not want to make any decisions that made it more likely that he would have to leave the home.

CHAPTER 3

Personalisation

Medicine is a land of heuristics: the learned fluency of experience manifests itself in the reverse parsing of presenting symptoms into a unifying diagnosis. Taken to it limits, the rapid identification of the patterns of presentation can confer the whiff of the godly to the practitioner – the subsequent worship is encouraged by way too many doctors. For what they are displaying is not genius but merely the nature of human learning, of finding patterns and rules, to reduce the need for a priori deductions with each new case.

Heuristics are good, but they are not infallible. A recent theme, for example, has been the focus on the rapid identification and treatment of sepsis, which improves survival. But there is a trap, which I'm sure you've spotted. Sadly, Matt Hancock, the then Health Secretary, didn't when he tweeted that death from sepsis is a 'preventable tragedy'.

The realm of heuristics in decision-making is a fascinating one: medical practice would often be impossible without them – there is simply too much work and too little time available to review, process and interpret all the data. Yet, their safe use depends on understanding their limitations. We are all prone to cognitive biases and each of us has biases that skew our thinking. The only way to counter them is to be aware of them. Jill Klein[1] outlines five pitfalls in medical decision-making: the representative heuristic (e.g. if a patient has biographical features typically representative of one illness, that illness is more likely to be diagnosed), the availability heuristic (diagnoses that come to mind easily are more likely to be made), over-confidence (this speaks for itself), confirmatory bias (we note features that confirm our initial expectations and ignore those that refute it) and illusory correlation (to perceive two events as related, whereas they are in fact entirely independent).

Wiser practitioners tend to be more muted and less bellicose in their prognostications. Confirmation bias exerts an insidious effect on the unwary, and the danger for all doctors is that they begin to believe their own hype. No matter how deep our empiricism goes, all the data we use to inform our practice tells us is the overall outcomes for a population of people: if the mortality rate for a procedure is 20%, how do we confer the risk appropriately to the patient in front of us? We have no way of knowing if they are one of the 20% or the 80%.

Balancing the limits of our knowledge with the need for the patient to have faith in their doctor is one of the more rewarding aspects of medical practice. It is based not just on what you 'know' but also on what you divine about the patient facing you. Much of the true meaning of medical advice lies less in the facts and figures and more in the sentiment and manner of the discussion. In an effective consultation, the doctor learns as much about the patient as the patient does about their condition. In geriatric medicine at least, there is a significant stylistic component to practice, and the style that should be emulated is that of the patient, not the doctor. This is the manner of the 'Mutual Participation' model, whereby the doctor and the patients act as equal partners in the relationship, sharing power, responsibility and knowledge.[2]

Sometimes, I am a struck by a preening sense of medical smugness – I have this warm glow that it is all going well. This is a dangerous time. Douglas Adams, in *The Meaning of Liff*[3] describes an 'Ely' as the 'first, tiniest inkling that something, somewhere has gone terribly wrong'. My warm fuzzy smugness is my own Ely – it is my bespoke heuristic, and as with other heuristics, it is never wrong, except for the occasions it is: '60% of the time it works every time'.[4]

Glibness and inattention are the scourge of the well-meaning medic. Being a good doctor for one patient is no guarantee of being a good doctor for the next patient, without the preservation of the approach that led to excellence. Good medicine is not ethereal – it is built on the predictable and teachable foundations of knowledge, empathy and good communication.

Health professionals have the advantage of experience over patients. Decision-making requires contextual familiarity, and it is this experience that helps us prepare patients for what comes next. A medical context is disarming: the emotional overlay in an otherwise technical and complex environment can prove overwhelming. Doctors are able to make decisions in high-pressured situations because they have lived the pressure to the extent that the situation itself is not novel – but they were not born that way; they learned.

For example, the first cardiac arrest I led was a planned shambles. By way of background, when a cardiac arrest call goes out in a hospital, the designated team rushes to the patient. It is usually the on-call medical registrar who 'leads' the call – it is their job to stand at the foot end of the bed and give instructions to each team member. They are specifically taught not to *do* anything – they think, they gather information and they instruct. A well-run cardiac arrest call is a thing of beauty – calm, efficient and without emotion.

I first led a cardiac arrest as a senior house officer when, on learning I had completed the Advanced Life Support course required to lead arrest calls, my supervising registrar told me that I would run the next one. It was a terrifying prospect. But when the time came, he stood behind me, watching what I was doing and making suggestions, and afterwards, he went through it with me. The next time an arrest call came round, there was none of the mystery and fear that had previously plagued me. It took me some time to become competent, but each time, I was better able to attend to the process rather than be distracted by the situation.

Often, the only way to learn how to deal with pressure is to experience it, parcel it up to one side and ignore it. If all you feel is pressure, you are not going to be able to focus on the steps you need to take to care for the patient.

When I have conversations with patients and relatives about serious or terminal diagnoses, it is as if they are leading their first cardiac arrest call. They are so smothered by their emotional responses to the situation that they cannot access their more rational selves to process the information and give instructions. In breaking bad news, the effective doctor brings their experience to bear on the situation – it is not so much the time for knowledge as the time for creating the environment in which questions can be posed and the first steps towards understanding are achieved. What patients and their relatives need from those moments is the space to attend to the matters that are important to them. By extension, there are some issues that their healthcare professionals need to attend to for them.

It is perhaps a temporary paternalism born out of the wish to allow patients the time to make effective decisions. The grip of powerful emotions can subvert usual reasoning, and it is the role of geriatricians, in particular, to create the time and space needed while delivering the best medicine possible. The patients' perceptions of success are influenced by the degree of agency that they are afforded in the decision-making processes.

In moments of crisis, patients respond variably: the patient who ordered me to stop talking when I told her that her scan showed 'something which is bad news' was telling me that she wanted to get on with the business of dying without being burdened by the mechanics of it. She went home and died there. Other patients want to know everything, see their scans, have second opinions and understand all the options. Most want to know what the diagnosis is, whether it can be cured and how long they have left – the rest they outsource to be managed on their behalf.

The only correct way to deal with patients is to be adaptable to their needs. An effective doctor translates the pathology the patient is experiencing into language they understand and adapts the treatment strategies to their particular goals and needs. Sometimes, the most important thing a doctor does is, to borrow a phrase, keep their head while the patient is busy losing theirs.

Some patients take a form of comfort in knowing that what is happening to them has happened to others, as if there is something grounding in finding out that you are not special. In this manner, their doctors and nurses form the continuity between their suffering and the suffering of others. Sometimes, all we do is bear witness, and that is often enough. The process of dying is a necessarily lonely one – as the guardian of knowledge about disease and death, there is only so far along the path that I can walk with them.

The mode of companionship towards death is an important role for healthcare professionals. Patients and families are often reassured by the efficient but gentle care of staff familiar with working at the edges of life. Through the process of medicalising death, however, not only has our collective familiarity with death been eroded, but so has our understanding of it. In our individual ignorance of death, we assume that what we don't know must be known by someone else. Yet death remains a process that we can only paint in outline – the details can only be coloured in after the event.

The healthcare profession, indeed the law of our land, is complicit in this: for every patient of mine that dies, I am obliged to give a cause of death. This perhaps derives from a general perception that ill-health is discrete and identifiable: it is simple, but sad, when a man drops dead from a heart attack or a woman succumbs to metastatic breast cancer, but the majority of deaths I encounter cannot be described in such detached terms.

We have seen before that humans fail the way any complex

machine fails – randomly and gradually. In practice, this presents as a sequence of seemingly individual but actually interconnected events, which Atul Gawande describes as, 'One damn thing after another.'[5] Frequently, there is a final illness that can be identified as the cause of death – pneumonia is still the 'old man's friend'. Yet, in distilling down the gradual and random failure of multiple human bodies to single final illnesses, we are embedding the lie that ill-health is episodic and discrete. Often, it is not, and, particularly in geriatric medicine, the truth that one has to acknowledge is that the patient started 'dying' well before they came under my care: as Elisabeth Kübler-Ross says, 'death is just a moment when dying ends.'[6] Life is a terminal diagnosis, and while medicine has smoothed out many of the historical troughs, it has not cured us of mortality.

Terminal illness is a compression of normal life: it shines a bright spotlight on the question that hangs over all of us of how we contend with our inevitable mortality. The modern bias to mortality is a combination of denial and control. The language of mortality is littered with value judgements around the use of words such as 'fight', 'brave' or 'battle'. If we frame life as a struggle then it is our Sisyphean task – we are bound to lose each time, forever.

One lie of modern medicine is that every health problem, and by extension our own mortality, is simply a technical exercise. We can see the same bias present in the collective inertia around dealing with climate change – we are waiting for a technological solution that will make redundant the need to look at our own lives. With mortality, as with climate change, it is not simply a matter of science, and yet popular discourse and daily medical consultations are littered with references to solutions, and cures, and action. As I write, we are in the middle of the first phase of the coronavirus pandemic. Society has been locked down, social distancing enforced, and we are wondering what happens next. There is the implicit assumption that biomedical sciences will develop a vaccine to protect us all, and the only question we are asking is when, not if. It may well be that a vaccine is technically possible (and you will know the answer by the time you read this), but once again, there is a focus on the technical solutions to the problem rather than the structural ones that have led to the current situation.

The question 'How long do I have left?' is one that doctors do well to swerve. The evidence suggests that doctors are poor at predicting the time left for patients in the final phase of life, and the better they know a patient, the worse their predictions.[7] The question itself can be viewed either as a function of the search for control in the face of overwhelming news or an emblem of the expectation that doctors today can give the certainty the patient seeks.

In reality, the question often misses the point, and discussions can be more usefully centred on the question, 'Now that you know you have limited time left, how would you like to spend it?' The details of death and dying are currently beyond our science, and I suspect they always will be. In fact, I suspect that it might be better for us if they always are. A brief thought experiment into immortality reveals the risks, not just of an ever-growing population, but also of the increasing accumulation of wealth to the wealthy and the immortal, as well as the suppression of meaning for younger people, perpetually excluded from personal progress due to the persistence of their forebears in the world ahead of them. More philosophically, it is mortality that gives us the potential to attend to personal meaning and impact, put in parentheses by the fact that we are here for only a brief time.

The relief of suffering and the eradication of illness are different outcomes. In the context of the reality that we are mortal, and we always will be, there is the need for balance to be struck between the pursuit of technical excellence in the care of old age, with the appreciation that a good old age is less a function of medical technology and more a function of spiritual and social satisfaction.

In the face of clinical futility, it is attention to spirituality that makes the biggest difference, as does the appreciation that death is, and always has been, a spiritual process. Spirituality can be understood without reference to religion, and in this context, it refers mainly to the human tendency to search for meaning. Ernest Becker describes the human condition as an unresolvable conflict between our mortal, fallible animal bodies and our immortal, abstract minds,[8] and says that those who die well, die without the need for 'symbolic identity' – which is to say that these are the people who understand that life is not all about them. It is his argument that human fear, of which fear of mortality is our most basic and fundamental, will always be spiritual, and it is why we grant figureheads immortality and why we bid for immortality through our actions or subscriptions to tribes, movements and religion. He ascribes much human behaviour (and he is not without his critics) to the quest for immortality in the light of the inevitable failure of our bodies. If one cannot live on in the physical, how does one live on in the abstract?

For much of our modern history, it is religion that has solved our spiritual need best, but this is down less to its 'truth' and more to its ability to commit us to a non-physical narrative of meaning and place in the world. If one accepts that the modus operandi of the human race has been the cooperation across distance and numbers through the aggregation around the shared narratives handed down to us, from mythology, origin stories and religion, then with it comes the understanding that we remain rooted in stories and, by design, sensitive to the power of stories regardless of how unhinged from fact they really are. It is a tendency that cannot be reasoned away – we are drawn to and compelled by a good narrative.

If one takes the microcosm of geriatric medicine in this context, one can begin to understand that while excellence in geriatric care is to some extent dependent on technical excellence and the appropriate application of best evidence, the holistic tenets of geriatric medicine invite us to consider the spiritual needs of our patients, particularly as they near the end of their lives. The nuances of individual beliefs and rituals are not amenable to shortcuts. It used to be simple – one would call for a priest to administer the Last Rites – but the waning of religion as a dominant social force has left greater variety and even a void where established rituals used to be. The individual response to imminent mortality is now more individual and less structured than ever before.

A challenge for geriatric practice is to embrace the absence of ritual, but rather than replace it with medical activity that distracts from the absence, have conversations that allow patients' personal meanings to be aired and final needs to be met. If we accept the persistence of mortality (either as a positive choice or a technical limitation), we ought to accept the challenge of attending to the needs of the imminently dying, beyond their presentation as a technical-medical exercise. Often, in practice, it is less the excellence of medical care that makes the difference to patients and their families at the end of life, but more the expression of human qualities: compassion, kindness and dignity mean an awful lot when one is dying. There is no mutual exclusivity between technical excellence and kindness, but there is an imbalance inherent in the systems that care for the dying in hospital, and a redress of this discrepancy is achievable, affordable and capable of delivering considerable benefits.

Endnotes

1   Klein, J. (2005) 'Five pitfalls in decisions about diagnosis and prescribing.' *British Medical Journal 330*, 7494, 781–783.

2   Szasz, T. and Hollender, M. H. (1956) 'The basic models of the doctor-patient relationship.' *AMA Archives of Internal Medicine 97*, 5, 585–592.

3   Adams, D. and Lloyd, J. (1983) *The Meaning of Liff*. London: Pan Books.

4   Apatow, J. (dir.) (2004) *Anchorman: The Legend of Ron Burgundy*. Dreamworks Pictures.

5   Gawande, A. (2014) *Being Mortal: Illness, Medicine and What Matters in the End*. London: Profile Books, p.208.

6   Kübler-Ross, E. (1969) *On Death and Dying*. New York: The MacMillan Company, p.254.

7   Christakis, N. A. and Lamont, E. B. (2000) 'Extent and determinants of error in physicians' prognoses in terminally ill patients.' *Western Journal of Medicine 172*, 5, 310–313.

8   Becker, E. (1973) *The Denial of Death*. London: Souvenir Press.

Simon

I often struggle to remember patients just by name. I see so many that they all merge into an indistinct haze. With a little thought, however, I can usually recall the details, but I have to find the right trigger. It is never the symptoms or the diagnosis that I remember first (my memory obviously isn't organised like that) but usually some key piece of biographical information – a story they told me, a comment they made or what job they used to do.

However, I have no trouble recalling Simon. He was younger than most of my patients (about 72). The approach to my office is down a long corridor, and as I stood at my door watching him draw near, I was struck by two things: the broad smile on his face and the broad gait with which he walked. Walking was clearly a very great effort for him. Using two sticks, he walked, or more accurately shuffled, towards me, with his legs splayed wide apart and leaning precariously forwards. His feet slid along the floor and then lifted horizontally before slapping down on the ground. The effort was palpable, concentration clear, but the smile was unbreakable.

One's instinct is to help, but he was determined and capable. I did not need to undermine him by helping him.

His problems had developed over the previous six months and his GP had assured him that it was simply the unfortunate consequence of advancing age. However, as his symptoms developed, the GP became less sure of the diagnosis and referred him to me.

Twenty years ago, I might have said that 72 was old – but I hope not. Today, it seems young. People do slow with age, but not as Simon had done.

Good practice in medicine is founded on knowledge, experience and accurate elucidation of the signs and symptoms on which to use that knowledge and experience. With practice comes fluency and with fluency comes familiarity. In the set of older patients I see, it is easy to spot what constitutes 'normal' and what is 'abnormal'. Simon's presentation was not normal.

Basing the degree of intervention on how he was when I first met him would have been dangerous. If you meet people when they are poorly, it can be difficult to imagine them when they are well. One can rapidly conclude that intervention would be futile. However, it quickly became clear that Simon had deteriorated a lot: six months earlier, he had enjoyed long walks with his dog and was an active member of lots of local community groups. He enjoyed none of those activities now.

To pare down a longer story, a CT scan of his brain revealed Normal Pressure Hydrocephalus. For reasons that are poorly understood, this condition causes an accumulation of the fluid that normally circulates around the brain and within its fluid-filled chambers within. As the cranium is rigid, the fluid build-up compresses the brain, causing neurological dysfunction, much like I saw in Simon.

After a delay of some months, a neurosurgeon fitted a tube from one of his ventricles (the fluid-filled chambers) to his abdomen. A pressure valve allowed the excess fluid in his brain to be siphoned off into his abdomen and prevented the brain from being squashed.

His walking never returned to normal, due to the permanent damage to his brain from the months of compression before his shunt was fitted. However, he can now be seen regularly out and about in town, always smiling.

CHAPTER 4

The Natural Limits of Medicine

In the last chapter, I drew upon the work of Ernest Becker,[1] who argues that while death is, and remains, our unavoidable destiny, our symbolic representation has moved away from participation in large, formal groups (particularly religion) towards individual, self-defined symbolic representation. Accepting the fact that the world will continue without us defies our self-view and confirms our unpalatable irrelevance; but as the saying goes, the graveyards are full of people the world could not do without.

The in-sourcing of individual purpose has been accompanied by parallel outsourcing of the mechanics and rituals of death to modern medicine. Overriding these changes is the emergent realisation that the absence of collective symbolic identify affirms the human bias to imagine our animal selves as immortal and abstract, resulting in our blind fumbling through life, too often blissfully self-deluding or in denial of our guaranteed mortality.

Reconciliation to mortality is a personal matter. It appears to be made easier by subscription to either formal religion or a social movement that makes promises about the afterlife or reassigns personal meaning to a wider whole. The modern way, however, seems to centre on blithe blinkeredness, which is one way of dealing with it, I suppose. The past can teach us something about the acceptance of mortality, but our approach need not be regressive. Progress can be garnered from the appreciation of our missteps and slight correction of the course we are currently on.

For example, we have created a faith in technology and scientific advance born out of the experience of watching our daily lives change rapidly and out of reckoning with the past; we have witnessed medical advances transforming the experience of a multitude of illnesses and all but eradicating a few. From these successes, we have both over-extrapolated the potential for modern medicine and misidentified dying and death as medical challenges to be dealt with as technical exercises. We have outsourced our understanding and familiarity of death to technical services, with an implicit blind faith that mortality is simply a technical problem in search of a solution.

In so doing, we have misunderstood the tenets of human nature and recast ourselves as a technological species, ignoring the millennia of history that characterise us much more consistently as spiritual beings with a predilection for stories. What defines our lives is not what we know but what we believe – an assertion that is confirmed in every walk of life, every day, and plays out with particularly macabre consequences in modern political discourse: the re-emergence of far-right movements, nationalism, anti-Islamic sentiments, Brexit, the rise of Donald Trump and our failure to react quickly enough to climate change all speak of our subscription to beliefs, not knowledge, and the outsourcing of our moral agency to technology rather than personal behavioural change.

Your disagreement on at least some of the arguments above is expected. It is offered without the intention to persuade (although the more the merrier with this particular view of atheistic, spiritual liberalism) but rather to give context to what follows. In any discussion about dying and death, your own approach will be necessarily informed by your spiritual identity.

Elisabeth Kübler-Ross points out that it is impossible for us to face death all the time – not as normal humans, nor as people with terminal diagnoses. She observes that denial is often, indeed usually, used by people on their path to acceptance. It constitutes a temporary defence, which allows people to continue to function even in the face of their own mortality. The need for denial varies but eventually wanes: those very close to death will tend to use isolation more than denial.

When I met Martin, he was a sprightly and engaging 94-year-old man with a penchant for wine gums. In the 30 years since he had retired, he had applied himself to cataloguing Dinky cars. He had given up driving a car the year before, when he was chastened by the news of a crash suffered by his 45-year-old neighbour. He had never had an accident, but he was self-aware enough to know that he was a local news headline waiting to happen. He sold his car and told me, 'I've spent the money, but I've no idea what on – all I know is that it's all gone.' He seemed rather excited by the recklessness.

Over the next 18 months, he pottered along. He never had any momentous medical problems, but there was the sense that his body was starting to fail: he fell over a couple of times, after which he went to hospital for brief admissions. After a hiatus of about a year, I saw him again at home, and the change was marked: he had taken to spending more and more time in bed, his appetite was poor, but perhaps most alarmingly, there were no wine gums to be seen. Also unnerving was the news that his Dinky catalogue was complete – leaving a gaping absence of purpose.

Martin found himself caught in a spiral of deconditioning: following his falls, he was more wary of walking around his house, which in turn led to further muscle wasting, worsened weakness and more risk of falls. The loss of his appetite was an ominous sign – it is often seen as people reach the end of their lives. He was not hungry, but he was bothered by being pestered by his children to eat more, so he started to fib about what he had eaten.

Martin fell again, and in his frail state, he fractured his hip. The process for patients with hip fractures is that there is no debating, no reasoning: they are taken to hospital where they have an operation to fix the fracture as quickly as possible. However frail or sick someone is, an urgent operation is the best way to manage their pain. However, a fractured hip is not so much a broken bone as it is a sentinel event: 30% of patients who have had a fractured neck of femur will be dead within a year.[2] It is often after the operation that the real work begins: a good recovery depends on rapid mobilisation of the patient to prevent excessive muscle wasting, which limits mobility. The muscle mass of older people must be protected, for the simple reason that once they have lost it, they find it difficult to exercise to the level required to build more.

Martin, however, proved reluctant to participate in exercises; he fatigued quickly and preferred to spend the day in bed with his hat on, either reading the newspaper or sleeping. In conversation, he would talk about his desire to recover and to return home. He would speak often and excitedly about how proud he was of his grown-up grandchildren, who by any conventional measure were doing very well. Yet, every aspect of his body language spoke of a man tired of life and ready to die. When asked directly if he wanted to recover, he would say that he was prepared to put in the work necessary to regain his mobility. He would talk about his desire to return home. When it was suggested to him that he came across as someone ready to die, he would look surprised and talk again about the motivation he drew from seeing his grandchildren do well. Yet not once would he agree to take part in a session with a physiotherapist or to spend much time out of bed. He continued to be dependent on the nurses for all his personal care, and in the end, when it became apparent that he would not regain mobility, he was discharged to a nursing home, where he died a short time later.

There was no conflict with Martin. Conversations with him were convivial, and he remained an engaging and bright conversationalist almost to the end. He expressed something a great many people in his position express – denial. He knew that he was dying, and in many ways, he was prepared for it. What he most regretted, however, was that he wouldn't live long enough to see just how well his grandchildren would do – this was so difficult to face up to that he found it easier not to face up to it at all.

Avery Weisman[3] suggests that denial is not a sign of unhealthy coping but rather a tool used by people to integrate reality at a pace they can manage. Often, patients will move in and out of denial, perhaps in the space of a single conversation, as they deny the parts they are most sad at losing or missing.

There is therefore a degree of circumspection required in supporting people in their dying days. I have no doubt that Martin knew he was dying, and I am sure he was ready for it. Even so, he was still very sad about not finding out how his grandchildren would do, and that was too much for him. One gained nothing by forcing him to confront the issue. No one could change it for him – it was a simple, unpalatable truth that had to be borne. All he needed was to be well cared for and to know that he could talk to us about anything, if he wanted, whenever he wanted.

Creating the conditions in which patients can face up to death well requires the alignment of several factors – those of the patient and the system looking after them – but it starts with the culture they exist in.

Our attitude to death and dying is a function of the values of the society and culture we live in. The way we care for older people reflects these values and derives from the manner of existence for older people in contemporary society. The discourse about death and dying in modern culture is skewed, affecting our perceptions of ill-health and even the mechanisms of death. Williamson and colleagues[4] showed that within mainstream media there is an over-representation of deaths from some cancers, 'flu and dementia and an under-representation of deaths from chronic obstructive pulmonary disease (COPD) and strokes. Also insidious is the language used in the context of illness: fight, battle, struggle, survival, hero.

These words all paint illness as adversarial. The average age at death is 80 years old.[5] The majority of people who die do not lose a battle; they reach the end of their run. Yet too often their route to a 'normal' death is framed in terms of a new illness that itself is characterised as something to be beaten. The general perception of life being a struggle against illness is something that filters through to the care of older people in a way that is unhelpful at best and harmful at worst.

In arming ourselves against illness with the best medicine available, we have started to lose our perspective. The typical route to terminality begins in some form of medical conversation, usually sought to achieve a cure. It is a wide statement, but within it is the essential (but not unarguable) truth that, today, it is doctors who decide if a problem is curable or incurable – if a patient is likely to live or die. It is doctors who assess, investigate, diagnose and determine what the treatment should, or could, be. The process of dying is understood in terms of the explanatory medical pathology causing the body to fail. It is, therefore, a function of medical practice to identify if someone is dying.

Yet the motivation of healthcare professionals is to diagnose and cure. And therein lies the tendency to attend to dying late. The modern characterisation is that death is what happens when medical science fails or reaches its limits. It is what happens when cures have been tried or when diagnosis evades our scanners and blood tests. Death is what happens when doctors fail. Yet clearly this is not right, for we all die.

The assessment of a frail person in ill-health takes place in the doctor's surgery, hospital clinic or inpatient ward. It is framed by all the biases of modern medical practice, which fundamentally reduce individuals down to discrete episodes of ill-health or individual long-term conditions, which are managed by protocol with too little reference to the other medical problems that person may have. Too often the knowledge that is brought to bear on the patient is medical knowledge rather than knowledge of the patient.

This bias and the relentless pressures on the health system have had a telling impact on the nature of medical services for older people: in the grip of rising numbers of older patients and tightened resources, health services have doubled down on managing the day-to-day strains on the system. This is most keenly felt by the patients being admitted through EDs and acute medical takes. Between 2003 and 2015, emergency admissions via EDs rose by 65%.[6] The result is that the practice of medicine in between episodes of ill-health has been scaled down; patients who would have previously been followed up in hospital clinics have been handed back to their GPs for ongoing management, but the number of GPs in practice has risen only slightly.[7] Geriatric medicine is not the holistic management of complex and frail patients over time that it ought to be; it is the practice of acute medicine in older people, which is something very different.

Thus, we find ourselves in a bit of a bind: the process of diagnosing and managing the issues in the run-up to death have been handed over, almost entirely, to medical services. However, those services are not necessarily best placed to meet those needs, both in terms of the cultural approach to dying and death, and due to resource problems in meeting the expressed need. There are, therefore, cultural and system issues that subvert the appropriateness of medical input to frail and older patients. These play out in the apparent focus on diagnosis and treatment in the short term rather than an understanding of individuals' needs over time that is both patient and holistic. The current health system is not designed for or adapted to managing the ill-health of old age that signals advanced senescence, because too much of the medical work takes places out of the context of that person's normal life.

It is natural that many aspects of the care of older people have been co-opted as part of healthcare provision – modern healthcare has delivered many benefits, but it is not a perfect fit. For instance, the model of care that older patients need is not simply a remoulding of the medicine applied to single illnesses in younger patients as a package deal. The interplay of multiple illnesses and multiple treatments creates significant complexities and risks that cannot be managed if each illness and its treatment is considered in isolation.

Furthermore, to consider the challenges of old age purely as medical problems is to take a narrow view of what old age is. The nature of any medical problem is modified by the presence of frailty, which renders individuals more liable to experience the pitfalls and complications of medical intervention and treatment. Frailty also creates a different landscape of expectation – one in which the expectations for medical intervention are necessarily more guarded. Yet the incorporation of 'frailty' as a medical diagnosis runs the risk of creating expectations for its treatment that cannot be met.

Healthcare professionals tend to operate with the defined parameters that we can label as 'medical practice', and there remain a great many decisions and actions outside of medical practice that are pertinent to how we care for older people. For example, liver specialists tend not to be experts in the treatment of alcohol addiction, even though the most effective treatment for liver cirrhosis is abstinence from alcohol. Likewise, healthcare professionals are not the arbiters of meaning and are not always best placed to consider the context of the current illnesses by which a patient is affected in the picture of that person's whole life. Medicine has taken the reasonable view of understanding illness in the framework of empiricism, pathophysiology, pharmacology and surgical intervention, but there is still a great deal about life and illness that lies outside of the domain of expertise in medical practice.

Illness is more prevalent in old age, but old age is not only a medical experience. There are many other facets to existence in later life, which are neither covered by nor accounted for in medical practice. Tackling, for example, the issues of social isolation and loneliness is important for the health of older people. Even to characterise these as public health issues is to dodge the ideal outcome. Once again, these are issues representative of the broader structural problems faced by wider society. Opinions will differ as to the underlying cause and solutions. Indeed, the changes that we can make as individuals are limited, but the first stage is to recognise the need.

Medical services for the older people should strive constantly for excellence, but our elders will only be content and fulfilled when we understand that good healthcare is only one element of good care. The big gaps in the discourse about ageing are inclusion and a forthright appreciation that a frail, old age is the best we have to look forward to: no one ages without ageing, unless they die young. We should aspire to old age, and in creating the best possible old age in our communities, understand that we are creating the best possible old age for ourselves.

The absence of an adapted role for seniors in normal society functions can be viewed as one example of the waning of effective communities in all parts of life. George Monbiot[8] argues that by enslaving ourselves to purely economic measures of success, we have lost sight of the factors that more accurately assess our collective contentment, and in our pursuit of economic progress, we have succeeded in breaking down our own communities to the extent that the social constructs that give people meaning and purpose have disappeared, leaving us disengaged, miserable and disenfranchised. Fritz Schumacher argued in *Small is Beautiful*[9] that it is the ease of travel that creates in all of us a 'footlooseness' that disengages us from our commitment to our communities.

There is a challenge for health services to respond more accurately to the individual biographies of older people in shaping treatment, as well as the need to allow for patients at the end of their lives to attend to their spiritual needs without medical processes becoming overbearing. However, the successful care of people towards the end of their lives is necessarily framed by the societal contexts in which they live. The needs of the dying will never be truly met if they remain only in the precinct of medical practice. Present in the modern attitudes to dying and death is a collective denial about the reality and certainty of mortality – this is one circumstance in which denial should be challenged.

A shift from the dominance of medical practice in the business of dying enhances the quality of care delivered by medical services to the older people by enabling a more detailed understanding of what success looks like and allowing medical intervention to accommodate where each person is in their own personal timeline and biography. At present, medical intervention is often framed by medically validated outcomes. A pneumonia is treatable and therefore tends to be treated. But a pneumonia in a woman with advanced dementia is different to the same illness in an 84-year-old man who still runs the local Rotary Club and looks after his great-grandchildren one morning a week.

It is as inappropriate to subject older people to the full might of our medical machinery as it is to deny them entirely. Fortunately, neither response is required. It is perfectly achievable to build services over time that understand and appreciate the needs and goals of our elders and are founded on a detailed knowledge of their medical background, social circumstances and psychological and functional biographies.

In later chapters, we will explore both the medical systems that could exist and, importantly, the social contexts that influence the nature of how we live with our elders.

Endnotes

1   Becker, E. (1973) *The Denial of Death*. London: Souvenir Press.
2   Lisk, R. and Yeong, K. (2014) 'Reducing mortality from hip fracture: A systematic quality improvement programme.' *BMJ Quality Improvement 3*, u205006.w2103.
3   Weisman, A. (1972) *On Dying and Denying: A Psychiatric Study of Terminality*. New York: St Martin's Press.
4   Williamson, J. M., Skinner, C. I. and Hocken, D. B. (2011) 'Death and illness as depicted in the media.' *International Journal of Clinical Practice 65*, 5, 547–551.

5   Office for National Statistics (2018) *National Life Tables, UK: 2015–2017*. Accessed on 8/2/2022 at www.ons.gov.uk/peoplepopulationandcommunity/birthsdeaths andmarriages/lifeexpectancies/bulletins/nationallifetablesunitedkingdom/2015to2017.

6   Maguire, D., Dunn, P. and McKenna, H. (2016) *How Hospital Activity in the NHS Has Changed Over Time*. London: The King's Fund. Accessed on 8/2/2022 at www.kingsfund.org.uk/publications/hospital-activity-funding-changes.

7   Rolewicz, L. and Palmer, B. (2019) *The NHS Workforce in Numbers*. London: Nuffield Trust. Accessed on 8/2/2022 at www.nuffieldtrust.org.uk/resource/the-nhs-workforce-in-numbers#4-what-do-the-shortages-look-like-for-staff-delivering-care-close-to-patients-homes.

8   Monbiot, G. (2018) *Out of the Wreckage*. New York: Verso Books.

9   Schumacher, E. F. (1973) *Small is Beautiful: Economics as if People Mattered*. New York: Harper and Row.

Joan

Joan made it clear she was fed up with being alive. She lived alone in a two-bedroom house and until her 90th year had enjoyed an engaging social life: there was her weekly bridge club and lunch in the garden centre with friends, and every weekend, her son would take her out in the car for a potter and a cup of tea by the sea.

Joan was not lonely. She was well loved and well cared for. She had simply reached a point where the effort of remaining alive was insufficiently rewarding.

Two months before I met her, her life had changed: discharged from hospital after a three-week admission, she was now unable to leave her house. She understood poorly what had happened to her in hospital, but she could feel the effects: she was breathless, listless and despondent. The rehab team had assessed her after discharge and moved her bed downstairs; the physiotherapist was haunted by seeing the risks Joan had taken when she attempted to go up the stairs. Carers visited twice a day to help her wash and dress in the morning and prepare for bed in the evening. Between care calls, she was alone. She still had visits, but she said to me, 'It's like a living bloody wake. They sit and stare at me and make awkward conversation. It makes me feel lousy.'

She started spending more time in bed, later reasoning that if she wasn't going to be doing anything, there was little point getting dressed at all. When I met her, she was dishevelled and lying in her pyjamas.

Joan was afflicted by two medical problems: COPD (emphysema) and depression. Like many of her generation, Joan had understood for a long time that smoking was normal, healthy even. Even their doctors had smoked. She had given up smoking some years ago, but the damage persisted. Each breath through her brittle, scarred lungs was ever less oxygenated than the one before, and her heart compensated by pumping harder to improve blood flow. In the later stages of chronic lung disease, the heart eventually starts to fail – from the effects of having to work harder to pump blood to decreasingly efficient lungs. After a while, it reaches a point when it can't sustain the effort. Heart failure compounds the breathlessness of the primary lung disease by allowing the failing lungs to waterlog. This leads to difficulty in lying flat (in the supine position, the fluid in the lungs spreads out through the lungs) and therefore poor sleep. It leads to weight gain from the retained water and weight loss from the permanent physical effort of breathing hard all the time. Joan was a de-muscled woman with swollen and wet lungs.

Her hospital admission had been precipitated by a bout of 'flu. She had been to her GP for her jab, but even though the strain she had contracted was one she had been vaccinated against, her immune system had failed to respond effectively to the vaccine. This is why it is so important for healthcare workers to be vaccinated every year: older people and those who are housebound do not contract 'flu from going out and about – they have it brought to them by people visiting them, who are often carrying the virus without symptoms. The infection had caused a secondary pneumonia, which further affected her breathing, and in the face of the strain of infection, her heart failed further, causing further fluid accumulation on her lungs. For the three weeks she was in hospital, she largely remained in bed, losing yet more muscle and with it her ability to walk even short distances. It was a good illustration of the cycle of deconditioning that blights the lives of the sick and frail.

Joan's immobility hit her hard emotionally. She missed her social engagements and quickly realised that she was unlikely to regain her physical strength. When something bad happens to you, it is normal to feel down about it. Depression happens when being down is the only way that you can feel – your sadness is independent of the external triggers. The science of depression, such as it is, argues that there is a resetting of brain chemistry to a steady state of sadness, and the medications for depression aim to restore a normal brain chemistry balance by preventing the breakdown of serotonin in the brain.

I have used antidepressants frequently in my patients, not because I have huge confidence in their effects but because it is all I have to offer. Many of my patients are unable to participate in the equally effective talking therapies because of cognitive impairment.

Joan agreed to take antidepressants, and she seemed to respond. Over the next couple of months, she appeared more engaged and positive in our conversations. She hadn't physically improved, but she seemed to be finding more interesting ways to pass the time. She seemed to accept that if she couldn't leave the house for social engagements, she could bring the social engagements to her home. She began to hold court: sat in her armchair, she would receive guests and chat to whoever happened to pop in.

Yet, something changed in the run-up to her birthday – I saw her last about four weeks before her 90th. She said something that I barely noticed at the time but later it jumped out at me. 'Doctor, I never thought I'd reach 90, and I don't think I am happy that I have.' That was it. I had no clue that the next time I would hear about Joan, someone would be telling me that the day after her 90th birthday, she was found dead at home, killed by an overdose of sleeping tablets she had slowly accumulated over the previous year.

CHAPTER 5

Assisted Dying

'What kind of doctor are you?'
'I'm a geriatrician.' I know an explanation is needed. It always is. 'I look after older people.'

'Oh.'

'In fact, it was the reason I studied medicine in the first place.'

'Oh.' Pause. Followed by one of two responses: 'I don't know how you do it,' or, 'Isn't that really depressing when they all die?'

I have had the conversation above countless times. These answers reveal a benign ignorance about what makes a career in medicine rewarding. I have an unrequited hope that just once someone will nod and express their understanding of the value or satisfaction of caring well for the older people. I should not have to justify myself. I should not have to explain that death at the end of a long life is a natural ending, that there is less of the loss and anguish of someone taken before their time. A bad death is a tragedy, a good one is a triumph. If you think there is something perverse in celebrating a good death, you probably have not witnessed a bad one.

Life is a thought experiment in futility. Medicine is only ever tinkering around the fringes, fighting the losing fight. Understanding this futility is grounds not for despair but for circumspection. Creating better deaths at the end of long lives is work that has its own value.

A bad death is one riddled with pain and anguish. It is often the emotional symptoms that cut the deepest. Medication and syringe drivers can salve the most troubling symptoms, but no drug can relieve emotional pain.

Few of my patients seem unprepared for death. Most face it rather calmly or at worst with resignation. It is the relatives who do not. This can be a function of being blinkered to reality or perhaps guilt when they learn the end is near: they overcompensate for their absence by demanding ever greater levels of intervention from healthcare staff. It is healthcare professionals who bear the brunt of internecine dysfunction.

One can observe in the very old an insidious form of fatigue, which is often accompanied by loss of appetite. If you ever want to know what a Pyrrhic victory is, watch a grown child chivvy their parent to eat more: they may succeed in increasing their calorie intake, but the cost to their relationship is significant and the benefit negligible. The parent is not dying because they are not eating, they are not eating because they are dying. The anorexia of old age is physiological, not a lack of willpower. It is more important to recognise what the loss of appetite says about the person without the appetite. It is a sign that should circle us back to the questions we now know to be the most important: what matters most to you, and what is the most important use of the time you have left?

Periodically, I am reminded that nothing I say is new. For instance, many of my patients do not need to be introduced to the idea of their own mortality: they have both recognised it and prepared for it. It is these people who tell me to end their lives. Most of them do it phlegmatically, straightforwardly. They don't expect me to do it, but they want me to know where their thoughts are. For the sake of clarity, I explain briefly the legal pitfalls of their request. The patient will often shrug in a manner of boredom and disdain, as if they had hoped, but did not expect, I would rise above their expectations. Their response reminds me of the way a cat will signpost its displeasure with a haughty turn of the head. Occasionally these conversations are underlined by a deep despair. These are the conversations that both need and take a lot more time. I cannot act on the desire to be dead, but I can seek to understand the thinking that leads to the conclusion that death is preferable.

When one is reconciled with imminent mortality, a form of impatience sets in. One sees it in relatives, who, when emotionally prepared for the death, experience a mounting sense of frustration that the thing they have steeled themselves for hasn't happened yet. The guilt is tangible until it is talked about openly. A more powerful form of impatience is seen in patients, who tend to be more vocal about their eagerness for it all to be over. We must remember, however, that we die in as many ways as we live. Not everyone is reconciled with life, and not everyone wants to die because they have finished living. Some people wish to die, for example, because there is nothing for them to live for.

Assisted dying is a tricky subject. It is thin ice; one must tread carefully. One must also allow for the odd misstep when people try to navigate their thinking through this topic – it is easy to go wrong. Feelings often run high, making open, non-prejudiced debate difficult. It is a matter about which no one can claim the objective truth but about which people are often passionate. We ought to allow for difference in how we enact our own views about assisted dying in life, but it is a hazardous field. The position I offer you today is to be debated and honed. It is not the site of my final stand.

Discussions about assisted dying require safe spaces to say out loud things you might later regret or disagree with. It is a matter about which it is difficult to land one's views fully formed. It is not a simple, binary issue, for there are layers and consequences. The denial of assisted dying by law creates victims – those who want it but are denied it. The permission of assisted dying by law would create different victims – those who don't want it but feel they must or ought to opt for it. We must decide where the balance between personal choice and control lies and where we wish the risk of harm to reside. This kind of calculus is only possible if we are able to discuss our views openly and frankly. There is no single correct answer.

Specifically, there is often a single issue relating to assisted dying that swings one's personal view. Religion is a prevalent reason for arguing against it. If you have a single issue that trumps all others in the consideration of this matter, does it represent a personal point of view or should it apply universally to everyone? We need to avoid imposing our own value judgements on others.

A majority view of assisted dying seems to be in favour of it. The National Centre for Social Research[1] reported that 93% of people surveyed approved of or wouldn't rule out doctor-assisted suicide. Such surveys are useful for giving a broad sense of how people feel about an issue, but they do not come close to providing the required depth of discussion on an issue this complex and charged.

Some fuss arose when the Royal College of Physicians (RCP) altered its stance from being opposed to assisted dying to being neutral, which means that they neither support nor oppose a change in the law.[2] Interestingly, the change in position followed an RCP poll in which the largest voting bloc opposed assisted dying but without a majority. The proportion in favour of assisted dying grew but still lay behind the group opposed (32% vs. 43%). I have some trouble interpreting this change of position: the numbers suggest a shift in the views of its membership but not enough to warrant a change in position. It seems to be a change that is reflective of the view that the RCP should not influence the debate but should instead reflect the views of the wider population. This is perhaps indicative of the waning influence of the Royal Colleges generally, but an informed debate about assisted dying rests on informed opinions about the limits and potential for current medical practice.

The assisted-dying debate usually filters into public awareness in the context of high-profile legal challenges about the right to die of individuals with progressive and incurable neurological problems, such as Diane Pretty and Debbie Purdy. These are compelling examples of the need for autonomy and control in the face of incurable or progressive medical problems.

However, legislation for a minority can have unintended consequences on the majority. For example, the majority of end-of-life scenarios play out in older and frailer people, which is an entirely different context for facing death. The criteria for terminality and futility apply equally to patients at the end of long lives and people with motor neurone disease, for example, but the context for death in old age is different. Assisted dying as a defiant act in the face of a brutal illness resonates with me. Assisted dying at the end of a long life, in the dying embers of frailty, does not.

The central issue is autonomy: on the one hand, the autonomy of a woman in her 50s with motor neurone disease is definitely enhanced by the potential for assisted dying. The same is not definitively true for an older person. Assisted dying makes sense as an affirmative action by someone in full command of their self-worth, dignity and autonomy. Assisted dying can only be an allowable pathway for someone who values their life and whose life is valued by others. In the absence of these features, it risks being subtly coercive, abusively neglectful and permissive of the abandonment of societal norms and expectations.

To an older person who feels unloved and burdensome, how can one ever control for the insidious coercion of not being wanted or not having meaning? Someone who has little joy, love or meaning in their life might well be justified in seeking assisted dying, but would we be right to allow it?

For assisted dying to be an affirmative action at the end of anyone's life, it must be made with the understanding that it would be OK not to go through with it. That is not the case for the many older people who feel as if they have lived too long, who believe that they can best help their families by not being there anymore.

When assisted dying is not an affirmative choice, it is inevitably a negative choice made by people whose existence is so devoid of meaning or value that they consider it better to be dead than alive. Frailty and senescence bring with them numerous challenges and hardships. Day-to-day life is difficult or uncomfortable. It is possible to consider frailty and advanced old age as medical problems, but it is not clear to me that this is appropriate. This book outlines a range of difficulties that arise as we age, but many of these difficulties are functions of how we as a society accommodate the physical, cognitive, functional, psychological and social aspects of age, not how we manage the medical aspects of old age.

Of particular importance is the appreciation that loneliness in advanced old age stems from decisions made about the nature of retirement at the latter end of our working lives. Medical problems may set the tone for daily life in old age, but they are not deterministic on their own. Extensive arthritis may cause pain. Heart failure causes breathlessness and reduced exercise tolerance. Dementia causes memory loss or personality changes. Equally important, however, are the subjective circumstances in which older people experience these symptoms, whose effect may be compounded and magnified by, for example, insufficient social care to keep older people clean, fed and watered, or the absence of social interaction, the feeling of being loved or meaningful daily activity to give them purpose. Suffering alone is degrees worse than experiencing the supportive embrace of community and family.

Loneliness and elder neglect are common and probably under-diagnosed. The Campaign to End Loneliness estimates that there are 1.2 million lonely older people in the UK,[3] while a systematic review in 2008 estimated that a quarter of vulnerable older people are, 'at risk of abuse and only a small proportion of this is currently detected'.[4] It is within this social milieu that one experiences abundant examples of patients who are denied care or who decline it, because they prefer to keep their personal resources to give to their children as inheritance. I have trouble, therefore, accepting that requests for assisted dying are not influenced by the environment for ageing that we provide.

We have created a society in which we amply demonstrate that we do not value enough the lives of our elders. Throughout this book, I try to demonstrate that there is room for optimism, but significant change is needed. The risk of introducing assisted dying into this matrix is to offer patients the ultimate out from a society that fails to value their existence at all.

A repeated argument against assisted dying is that it will distract from investment in end-of-life care.[5] Disability commentators have expressed their nervousness at the prospect.[6] Countries that have legalised assisted dying have reported no problems with coercion, but how would one even prove it? Yet there does not have to be coercion for decision-making to be skewed. People who are concerned at the implications of assisted-dying legislation for them (e.g. people with disabilities) are amplifying wider concerns they face in their lives, namely that the potential for euthanasia gives a name to a mechanism that could be used to further exclude them from society. It is the fact that the prospect itself is a concern that should give us pause for thought: it is very unlikely indeed that anyone would be made to request assisted dying, yet marginalised groups feel as if they may be further marginalised by legalising it. That is a message we should attend to, because it points to something that, in our gilded, included lives, we are unaware of. In the absence of inclusion, or being cared for, assisted dying might become the only solution that some people feel is open to them. Even without coercion, it becomes the coercive inevitability of a society that does not care enough. It becomes not affirmative but reductive and negative.

The balance of the assisted-dying debate in this framing, therefore, is between assisted dying as a positive choice and as a negative one. Which way does the pendulum swing? In terms of absolute numbers, it swings towards it being a negative choice: the number of people to whom it might apply is higher among those with frailty. Indeed, the negative context to which I allude may be deepened by enacting assisted-dying legislation.

If we as a society consider assisted dying to be an important choice for individuals to have, it can only work as part of a package of societal reform that seeks to provide not just good care but also good inclusion in community life for older and frailer people. There is a long way to go before we have a society that values the contribution of the older people to everyday life and successfully includes them in its rhythms and routines.

That is the price for assisted dying.

Endnotes

1 National Centre for Social Research (2019) *My Death, My Decision: Campaigning for a More Compassionate Approach to Dying.* Accessed on 8/2/2022 at www. mydeath-mydecision.org.uk/wp-content/uploads/2019/03/Briefing-on-NatCen-assisted-dying-poll.pdf.

2 Royal College of Physicians (2019) 'No majority view of assisted dying moves RCP position to neutral.' Accessed on 8/2/2022 at www.rcplondon.ac.uk/news/no-majority-view-assisted-dying-moves-rcp-position-neutral.

3 Campaign to End Loneliness (n.d.) 'The facts on loneliness.' Accessed on 8/2/2022 at www.campaigntoendloneliness.org/the-facts-on-loneliness.

4 Cooper, C., Selwood, A. and Livingston, G. (2008) 'The prevalence of elder abuse and neglect: A systematic review.' *Age and Ageing 37,* 2, 151–160, p.151.

5 Godlee, F. (2019) 'Assisted dying: The debate continues.' *British Medical Journal 364,* 1576.

6 Campbell, J. (2019) 'Disabled people like me fear legal assisted suicide: It suggested that some lives are less worth living.' *BMJ Blogs.* Accessed on 8/2/2022 at https://blogs.bmj.com/bmj/2019/02/06/disabled-people-like-me-fear-legal-assisted-suicide-it-suggests-that-some-lives-are-less-worth-living.

Jack and Fanny

There are a number of benefits to seeing patients in their own homes: it is usually easier for me to travel to them rather than the other way around; it is less stressful for them too. I have seen people in clinic who were washed, dressed and sat by the front door hours before hospital transport was due to pick them up. This means that by the time they see me in clinic, they are tired and either desperate for the loo or desperate for a drink having not imbibed anything because they did not want their bladder to catch them short. However, the most compelling reason is accuracy: a patient in their own home tends to be less stressed, more honest and more natural. In clinic, they can dress up and pretend to me they are managing OK. Digging through what a patient thinks I want to hear to find the truth is a difficult skill. In their own homes, there is no disguising reality.

When I visited Fanny in the room of the residential home she shared with her husband, I was struck immediately by how clean and tidy the flat was but most of all by how well she was. This was surprising, because I knew that she had advanced dementia. Via the GP, the residential home had complained that she was difficult to manage. She was prone to emotional outbursts and, occasionally, physical aggression. It was my job to see what could be done.

Doctors are given privileged access to people's lives: we can ask questions that no one else would dare to ask, and more often than not we are given answers. Yet, for all our access, we only ever see briefly into people's lives and it is impossible to observe accurately all the relevant experiences in a single assessment.

Fanny spoke vividly about her past – she talked with fondness about meeting her husband and bringing up their children. She recounted wistfully the story of their road trip around Europe with their young family in the 1950s. However, any questions about the recent past or the present befuddled her. The mounting frustration was visible and she would frequently explode with vengeful statements, 'Stop asking such stupid questions!'

It was at these moments that her husband would step in, both defusing the tension and providing the answers. Jack was not just dutiful in attending to Fanny's physical needs but also adept at riding the tides of anger that erupted whenever her irritation boiled over. He was endlessly patient and unwaveringly kind in a way that even Fanny recognised. It had become her habit to call for Jack the moment she struggled with anything.

Keeping Fanny clean was no small task. She frequently soiled herself and he cleaned her up. Occasionally he would call for help from the staff, but he bore the bulk of the responsibility. Her cleanliness on my visit was not a one-off effort for my benefit: he was clearly in the habit of maintaining standards.

Looking around the small, two-roomed flat, I could see the small kitchen at one end of the living area, but I could not see a washing machine.

'Who does the laundry?' I asked.

'Well, the home does Fanny's but I do my own,' he replied.

'How?'

'In the sink, with washing-up liquid.'

It turned out that Fanny's behaviour had deteriorated because she had developed a rash that was irritating her. It was caused by the washing powder that the home was using to do her laundry.

My advice to them was to use non-biological powder and perhaps to do his laundry while they were doing hers.

CHAPTER 6

A Glimpse Beyond the NHS

It can be tempting to view the difficulties of the NHS purely as issues of demand and funding. It is difficult to refute the idea that the NHS has been in crisis-response mode over the past ten years, and it was in the context of this corroded resilience that the pandemic landed. The result is a deeply injured health service. Historically, NHS funding has increased by an average of 4% per year.[1] Since 2009, however, the average funding has increased annually by only 1.2%.[2] In that time, there have been significant changes in the nature and needs of the people served by the NHS. For example, ED attendances have risen 22% since 2008.[3] In 1991, over-65s comprised 15.8% of the population.[4] The ONS estimates that by 2041, they will account for 26% of the population.[5] In Dorset, where I used to work, that level has already been reached. At the same time, both the technology that can be brought to bear on illness and the expectations of patients have risen, expensively. Through the prism of an oversimplified history, one can assert that the NHS was formed at a high point of social cohesion and collectivism, yet we now find ourselves debating the function and needs of our health service at a time of entrenched social divisions and perhaps even selfishness. List to yourself the issues that divide us. Now counterweight them with the issues that unite us. Which way do your scales fall?

The nature of the demand on the NHS is also imperfect: NHS England reports that ED attendances for people aged over 60 rose by two-thirds between 2007/08 and 2013/14[6] – a rise that cannot be explained by demographic changes alone. It may well be the case that people are now living with medical problems that previously would have killed them, but it is equally possible that other factors contribute to the sub-optimal long-term management of their underlying conditions, which, in the absence of services in the communities that could meet their needs, results in their presentation at hospital. We also need to be wary of our faith in the objectivity of medical diagnoses and the presentation of ill-health. During the first lockdown, we saw low levels of non-coronavirus illness, suggesting that people were either not feeling unwell, not getting unwell or not seeking help when they needed it. As restrictions have lifted, demands on the health service have soared. Anecdotally, colleagues report to me that patients are both presenting later with more severe problems and presenting with simple problems that they may previously have managed themselves.

The purpose of this point is to emphasise that we should not oversimplify complex behaviours and should also understand that the NHS is not always used by people who either need hospital care or have problems for which a medical response is required.

It is easier to access the NHS than it is to access other forms of support, so it should be no surprise that many problems find their expression in medical terms, when in other systems and other countries, a different expression might be seen. The result is, or has been, that the health service has found itself under relentless pressure to meet expressed demands.

The experience of patients across the NHS has been affected by the reality of rising demand in the face of tightened resources,[7] but there is also the suggestion that more insidious forces are at play. The daily lives of staff working across the health service are blighted by the experience of working at full capacity, all of the time.

Burnout is an increasing risk for healthcare staff[8] and a function as much of organisational factors (such as workload, unpredictability, loss of control and an inability to influence the shape of one's job) as individual ones.[9] At least some of the capacity to weather the routine stresses of working in healthcare derives from the understanding that one's input is valued. However, the duration of the austerity-driven pay restraint in the NHS has continued for long enough for it to feel more like a statement of value than necessary cost saving. The British Medical Association (BMA) argues that between 2005 and 2015, doctors' real-term earnings fell by 22%.[10] If the sustainability of the NHS is dependent on the discretionary effort of the staff delivering the service, the climate of provision ought to seek to maximise that discretion. Failing to increase earnings in line with inflation inevitably sends the message to staff that their work is valued less than it used to be. Perhaps there is an assumption that the privilege of being a healthcare professional ought to be enough to sustain staff, regardless of how trying working conditions are.

The goal is not to start an austerity bun fight but merely to outline the semantic paradox that seems to taint the current discourse on healthcare – namely, that while we profess to care, our collective actions suggest that, in fact, we do not. A recent survey identified the NHS as the 'British' institution of which we are most proud.[11] Although public satisfaction has waned in the wake of performance problems, it remains high.[12] The key issue is not that older people do not have medical problems and do not require medical support but rather that the relative predominance of the description of the problems of ageing in medical terms and the accessibility of services through the NHS create a disproportionately large role for medical services for older people when they should ideally form one part of a holistic system for managing and supporting the aged as part of the routine operation of an inclusive society.

At its heart, the NHS was an ambitious socialist enterprise that embodied the understanding that illness is bad luck and our ability to ride the vagaries of fortune is enhanced by clubbing together. The UK has not been a socialist country in my lifetime (New Labour hardly counts) but the NHS stands as more than just the socialist delivery of healthcare. Until recently, the Commonwealth Foundation ranked the NHS as the best overall health system in the world.[13] Yet while it has always scored well for access, efficiency and equity, it performs poorly for outcomes. We can be proud to have a healthcare system that is efficient, accessible and fair, but we should also want a healthcare system that delivers the results we want.

The provision of healthcare is mired in political ideology. It is perhaps an inevitability of the state provision of a total healthcare service. However, there is at least a sense in which the NHS goes beyond simply being an effective means of funding comprehensive healthcare to a population and becomes an emblem of what we as a society are capable of at our very best. In that way, the NHS stands as an emotional and ethical surrogate for our own values and actions: having a health service that is free at the point of use and based on need rather than the ability to pay is our established model of care. It requires nothing of us now, except our continued contribution to the tax to pay for it. Its continuation, therefore, constitutes business as usual but allows us to feel as if we are each invested in the collective good. It is an achievement from the past that reflects well on the attitudes of the present.

What happens, however, if we jump down from the shoulders of the past? Evidence of the values and ambitions in which the ideals of the NHS were gestated become harder to find. A ten-year programme of politically motivated austerity has reset the expectations of what government, and society in general, should do for its most vulnerable. Older people and those with frailty are a subset of the totality of need in modern society, but the enacted practices for managing vulnerability have taken a hit so large that even an institution as large and as efficient as the NHS cannot mask the general underlying trends.

Wherever one looks, one finds a dilution of the practices of a modern, western democracy that protect the access to health, education, work and even justice. The domains in which we have traditionally pooled resources to afford a higher average standard than would be affordable individually have been pared back to the extent that those who have the means purchase the difference, while those who don't make do with what they are offered. For example, the Secret Barrister[14] paints a chilling picture of the restriction to justice for those accused of crimes: the availability of legal aid has been cut back as part of the austerity programme such that those who are accused of crimes are forced to either represent themselves (which has its own pitfalls) or exhaust all their funds and assets to defend themselves. If they are acquitted, they have little recourse to reclaim the costs incurred and are often bankrupted by the process of proving their innocence. Does that constitute justice?

A cursory look at all of the public institutions provided for the greater good reveals a parlous state of affairs: police funding has been cut by 20%,[15] local authorities' funding reduced by 49%[16] and benefits squeezed, and schools' funding has fallen 8% in real terms.[17] This is an indicative rather than comprehensive summary – to give a context for the consideration of our health service.

The justification that austerity was necessary to allow the government to balance its books was based on the disingenuous comparison of government debt to household debt. They are clearly not the same thing. One can only conclude that austerity was driven either by ideology or bad economics. There should be no problem with a policy underpinned by a consistent ideology, but that is not what we were given. Austerity was ideology masquerading as economic practice. It was, in fact, a simple assertion that the role of government needed to be scaled back and replaced by the Big Society, which was feted as social solidarity meets free market theory. The landscape of community cohesion required for the Big Society to work was, by definition, our problem.

The fate of public services over the last ten years is a deliberate plan to reduce the role of government in our daily lives. That by itself is not a problem; it is a perfectly valid position to adopt. It would also be disingenuous to categorise it simply as a function of the Conservative government: this is the party that we have repeatedly returned to government (to a greater or lesser extent), using the non-representative voting system that we chose to keep in the Alternative Vote referendum in 2011.

The important consideration that comes out of the brief diatribe above is the logical conclusion that we exist in a society in which it is implied that we seek a smaller role for the state and expect individuals and communities to create the services that once we relied on the government to provide.

Yet the rollback of government has happened with a speed and lack of transparency that leave us unprepared for what comes next. In order for communities to organise and rally around the local needs, they should have the means and resources to do so. Yet it is the structures and functions of communities that have been hit the hardest by austerity, in the parts of the country most in need of them. A Unison audit[18] paints a bleak picture of reduced neighbourhood police teams, closed libraries, youth centres and children's centres and reduced home care provision.

While a capitalist discourse dominates our understanding of what is important, we are in danger of embarking down a route of irreversible changes that state clearly that the value of everything is determined by its price, or the money that can be wrung out of it. Emblematic of this was *The Guardian*'s report in April 2020 that outlined that while the privatisation of the Forestry Commission was stalled in 2010 on the back of public reaction, the Commission has now developed proposals to allow for the development of chalets on its land, 30 sites at a time, with no upper limit on total development.[19] As ever, the devil is in the detail, but there is also something tainted in the headlines. Should we live in a world where a forest is valued for the money that can be made from it, or should we live in one in which forests are valued for simply being forests?

The impacts of our political choices are dramatic. The pursuit of austerity has distracted us from the key actions that make a difference to our health and welfare. The Institute for Public Policy Research estimates that our collective lack of investment in public health has resulted in 130,000 preventable deaths in the last seven years.[20] That in itself represents a missed opportunity, but there is also something important and more abstract in play: there is the emergence of an 'I'm alright Jack' philosophy, which implies that bad things only happen to the deserving and places the emphasis on self-determinism to raise our individual living standards. It's a rather selfish position to take but not in itself indefensible. What really grates is the emergence of a world in which no amount of honest endeavour can improve the lives of vast sections of society.

A prerequisite for a self-improving, industrious society is one in which social mobility is a lived reality. Let's not kid ourselves for a moment. The government's own Social Mobility Commission confirms that the key determinant of how well any child fares in life is a function of the affluence of the family they are born into.[21]

There is, therefore, much to ponder about the state of our society today. As a way of dispelling the gloom, try casting around for collective achievements from the last ten years that we can be proud of. Are you feeling better? Me neither.

There are few instances to hold up as examples of the UK as an ambitious, enterprising nation, seeking improvements in quality of life for its citizens. It is this context that is everything for the NHS. Even before one considers intergenerational conflicts that further taint our social dynamics, we have a health service that we say we value while continually failing to invest in it. We embrace the needs-based, centrally funded universal system for health but not for social care.

In that way, the NHS is itself the outlier in contemporary society. It is the modern institution that fits least well with the expressed values of the present. I once described the NHS as, 'a forward-thinking vision of the future from the past'.[22] In the matrix of public services that sit outside health, the NHS reflects the values and decisions of the past and is itself affected by the prevalent attitudes of the present.

If the ambition and values that created the NHS were driving forces today, there would certainly be a different resolution for social care, for example. For instance, The 'Dilnot Report',[23] highlighted that an individual's future social care costs were unpredictable and potentially unlimited, making them an uninsurable risk. The solution that Andrew Dilnot proposed was for us to pool risk, limit our maximum individual liability and use the state to step in for catastrophic care costs. It was a fair and relatively simple solution – there were associated costs, estimated at the time at £1.7 billion, and eight years later it still has not been implemented.

Below the headline that your future social care needs are your problem alone, the lack of action on social care funding plays out every day in the NHS. Having received all manner of investigations and treatments without reference to money, patients and their families have to learn quickly that the care they need to support them at home is not funded in the same way. In fact, the difference could barely be starker: a ruthless form of means testing asserts that anyone with funds over £23,250 must pay for their own care. Plans have recently been tabled by the government but stop well short of a fair resolution: wealthier homeowners remain less liable than poorer ones.

The transition from NHS-funded care to social care is abrupt and distressing, particularly for patients but also for staff, who bear the brunt of the anger and frustration at the inequity of the system. The issue of fairness is not so much about the requirement to pay but the role that luck plays. It is bad luck to require a large package of care in your old age. It is unpredictable and cannot be planned for. The risk cannot be insured against. A further inequity appears when people who have savings, either through good luck or hard graft, realise that all they have earned is the right to spend their money on their care. It's a realisation that leads to anguish and hurt, but it also gives rise to more deceitful practices.

For example, a patient with advanced dementia was forced to remain in hospital for months, because his daughter, who had a Lasting Power of Attorney for his financial affairs, refused to release his funds to pay for a care home. She was unusually honest about her reasons, stating that it was her view that the state should pay for him and the money that her father had saved should be for her. Most people have the courtesy to at least pretend that greed is not their driving motivation. This kind of attitude is prevalent, and it is a thread of this book that such behaviour is an inevitability of a society that encourages us all to think about our own welfare to the exclusion of the common good, and one in which our moments of misfortune are ours alone to deal with and not a problem for wider society.

It is the apparent incompatibility of the founding tenets of the NHS with the rules and standards of wider society that creates one significant existential threat to the NHS. As a final outpost of social solidarity, the compassion and goodwill of healthcare staff is eroded daily by routine unkindnesses that they are expected to both overlook and compensate for. The discharge plans of older patients are routinely delayed by families who do not want their relatives to spend their own money on their own care. The inequity of the social care system is difficult to refute, but more distasteful still are the plans that relatives have for the money they have yet to inherit. The neglect and abuse of older people is common yet attracts nothing like the attention of the same abuses in children.

There is a broader issue at play, which is illustrated by the nature of our social welfare structures: the transition to Universal Credit has not just simplified the welfare system but also firmly embedded conditionality as a requirement for receiving benefits.[24] In order to claim benefits, people must spend time looking for work, attend mandatory appointments or accept jobs found for them. Failure to comply can result in the halting of payments. The principle seems to be divorced from the implementation, and it is difficult to resist the conclusion that, by design, compliance is difficult to achieve. The positive impact of conditionality is unclear and public support for it varies.[25] However, it also speaks to a wider issue of individual rather than collective responsibility: failure to comply with the conditions imposed by Universal Credit and experiencing a reduction in funds can be framed as an individual responsibility rather than a collective one. For reasons that will be discussed later, it is difficult to expect from benefits recipients, who may be stressed by poverty and undermined by any number of experiences that limit their personal effectiveness, the same level of compliance and organisation that we would expect from someone in well-paid employment. We don't have a welfare system that accounts for behaviours and circumstances that inevitably limit the ability of people to navigate complex systems, and we don't have a benefits system that seeks to lift these people up. Instead, it appears designed to limit our collective liabilities towards these people, leaving them both impoverished and, perhaps more toxically, permanently insecure.

This perhaps is illustrative of a wider social trend, namely that we have embraced Mammon or perhaps forgotten that individual success is not built only on the success of individuals and there are important, non-monetary benefits to collective risk-sharing and support.

For example, I have been caring for a 96-year-old man with advanced prostate cancer that has spread to his bones. He is in terrible pain most of the time but has been reluctant to receive our help because he does not think he deserves it. Every time one of us visits him, he questions why we are wasting our time with him and not looking after younger (and therefore more deserving) patients. He suffers from a bias against older people and the vulnerable that he divines in his daily life, which derives from our consideration of ourselves as a collection of individuals rather than a closer-knit community.

Our health service will inevitably reflect the values of the society it serves. It is, after all, staffed and run by ordinary members of the public performing professional acts of kindness and care. Yet, their resilience is not limitless. The succour and satisfaction gained from caring for the sick and the vulnerable is offset and eroded by the relentless pressure of performing the same roles, at ever greater intensity, within a community that has begun to take you for granted, where criticisms and complaints become as frequent as thanks. In my own practice, I have noticed a trend over the last few years for formal complaints to come not from my patients themselves but their relatives – often people who were little present either in the period before or during the patient's hospital admission. I cannot pretend that our care is always perfect – we make mistakes – but I can place alongside that admission the observation that blaming health services for unwanted outcomes sometimes acts as a substitute to the personal blame of the person making a complaint. The services to whom the responsibility of caring for elders has been outsourced are also blamed when things go wrong. Advocacy has replaced direct care and compassion as the unit of filial responsibility.

The ability to care is not limitless, but it can be replenished by the appreciation that the act of providing care or treatment is only one part of a wider culture of taking the needs of its citizens seriously. If we applied the attitudes of the NHS to education, social care, community resources and public health, we would no longer need to hold the NHS up as our proudest achievement – it would simply be a reflection of the way we do things.

The NHS is a brilliant way of delivering healthcare. It provides levels of efficiency and equity unrivalled in the world,[26] but it shines a light on the extent to which we collectively fail to invest in each other. Thus, the secret to ensuring that our most frail citizens are well looked after begins with the appreciation that the solution does not lie in the health service – it lies in social care, community resources, public health endeavours and the general understanding that everyone benefits if we pool our resources and talents for the collective good.

It would take volumes of work to articulate appropriately all of the issues relevant to this topic. However, the message should be that how we provide healthcare and care for the vulnerable and older people is as much a function of how we conduct ourselves generally as it is of the structures and processes of health and social care. We have the health and social care systems we deserve because each exists in the form it does from the collective choices we have made politically and socially – and each has been funded to the level that we consider appropriate. Deficiencies in either structure or funding represent deficiencies in the levels to which we value them. In this way, the systems we have are a mirror of the society in which we live: if we do not like what we see in the mirror, we should not shout at the reflection looking back at us.

Endnotes

1   The King's Fund (2018) *The NHS Budget and How it Has Changed.* London: The King's Fund. Accessed on 10/2/2022 at www.kingsfund.org.uk/projects/nhs-in-a-nutshell/nhs-budget.

2   *Ibid.*

3   NHS Digital (2018) *Hospital Accident and Emergency Activity, 2017-18.* Accessed on 10/2/2022 at https://digital.nhs.uk/data-and-information/publications/statistical/hospital-accident--emergency-activity/2017-18.

4   Office for National Statistics (2018) *Living Longer: How our Population Is Changing and Why it Matters.* Accessed on 10/2/2022 at www.ons.gov.uk/peoplepopulationandcommunity/birthsdeathsandmarriages/ageing/articles/livinglongerhowourpopulationischangingandwhyitmatters/2018-08-13#how-is-the-uk-population-changing.

5   *Ibid.*

6   NHS England (n.d.) *Improving Care for Older People.* Accessed on 10/2/2022 at www.england.nhs.uk/ourwork/clinical-policy/older-people/improving-care-for-older-people.

7   NHS England (2019) *Statistical Press Notice: NHS Referral to Treatment (RTT) Waiting Times Data*. Accessed on 10/2/2022 at www.england.nhs.uk/statistics/wp-content/uploads/sites/2/2019/03/RTT-statistical-press-notice-PDF-559K-89382.pdf.

8   Imison, C. (2018) *Addressing Staff Burnout: A Moral and Ethical Imperative*. The Nuffield Trust. Accessed on 10/2/2022 at www.nuffieldtrust.org.uk/news-item/addressing-staff-burnout-a-moral-and-ethical-imperative.

9   Lemaire, J. B. and Wallace, J. E. (2017) 'Burnout among doctors.' *The British Medical Journal, 358*, j3360.

10 British Medical Association (2021) *BMA Demands DDRB Recognises the Value of Doctors*. Accessed on 10/2/2022 at www.bma.org.uk/collective-voice/influence/key-negotiations/doctors-pay/annual-pay-review-from-the-ddrb.

11 Mintel (2018) *British Lifestyles: The NHS Tops List of UK's Most Cherished Institutions*. Accessed on 10/2/2022 at www.mintel.com/press-centre/social-and-lifestyle/british-lifestyles-the-nhs-tops-list-of-uks-most-cherished-institutions.

12 Robertson, R. (2019) *Why Is Public Satisfaction with the NHS Still Falling?* London: The King's Fund. Accessed on 10/2/2022 at www.kingsfund.org.uk/blog/2019/03/why-public-satisfaction-nhs-still-falling.

13 The Commonwealth Fund (2021) *Mirror 2021: Reflecting Poorly*. Accessed on 10/2/2022 at www.commonwealthfund.org/publications/fund-reports/2021/aug/mirror-mirror-2021-reflecting-poorly#rank.

14 The Secret Barrister (2018) *The Secret Barrister: Stories of the Law and How it's Broken*. Picador: London.

15 Maguire, P. and Chakelian, A. (2018) 'The deepest cuts: Austerity measured.' *The New Statesman*. Accessed on 10/2/2022 at www.newstatesman.com/politics/uk/2018/10/deepest-cuts-austerity-measured.

16 *Ibid.*

17 Tighe, C. (2019) 'UK councils "on life support" as lack of funding takes its toll.' *Financial Times*. Accessed on 10/2/2022 at www.ft.com/content/f89022a2-2fab-11e9-8744-e7016697f225.

18 Unison (2015) *An Austerity Audit: Coalition Cuts to Local Communities in England since 2010*. Accessed on 10/2/2022 at www.unison.org.uk/content/uploads/2015/05/On-line-Catalogue23139.pdf.

19 Jenkins, S. (2018) 'Will we stand by and watch the privatisation of our forests?' *The Guardian*. Accessed on 10/2/2022 at www.theguardian.com/commentisfree/2018/apr/27/privatisation-forests-forestry-commission-commercial-development.

20 Helm, T. (2019) 'Austerity to blame for 130,000 "preventable" UK deaths – report.' *The Guardian*. Accessed on 10/2/2022 at www.theguardian.com/politics/2019/jun/01/perfect-storm-austerity-behind-130000-deaths-uk-ippr-report.

21 Social Mobility Commission (2019) *Social Mobility in Great Britain – State of the Nation 2018 to 2019*. Accessed on 10/2/2022 at www.gov.uk/government/publications/social-mobility-in-great-britain-state-of-the-nation-2018-to-2019.

22 Dharamshi, R. and Hillman, T. (2013) *Today's Service, Tomorrow's System*. F20 Finnamore Essay Prize.

23   Commission on Funding of Care and Support (2011) *Fairer Care Funding: The Report of the Commission on Funding of Care and Support*. Accessed on 10/2/2022 at https://webarchive.nationalarchives.gov.uk/ukgwa/20130221130239/http:/dilnotcommission.dh.gov.uk/files/2011/07/Fairer-Care-Funding-Report.pdf.

24   Abbas, J. (2017) *Working Hard or Hardly Working? Universal Credit and the Problem of Conditionality*. Accessed on 10/2/2022 at www.england.nhs.uk/ourwork/clinical-policy/older-people/improving-care-for-older-people.

25   Abbas, J. and Jones, K. (2018) *In-Work Conditionality Is Based on Weak Evidence – but Will the Policy Sink or Swim?* Accessed on 10/2/2022 at https://blogs.lse.ac.uk/politicsandpolicy/in-work-conditionality-public-opinion.

26   Robertson (2019).

Roger

Roger suffered recurrent bouts of abdominal pain, triggered by constipation, low fibre, spicy foods and insufficient fluid intake. As a result of previous abdominal surgery for bowel cancer, he had developed scar tissue within his abdomen, called adhesions, which had a tendency to cause the bowel to kink and twist, resulting in bowel obstruction. His obstruction always relieved itself, but it caused him a lot of pain. Over time, we had established a regime of laxatives to both stimulate his gut and soften his poo to prevent further problems.

Roger's precise underlying pathology was not standard, but constipation is a common problem for older people. They drink little, causing their stools to harden, and they move little, causing the gut to slow down. Geriatricians talk a lot about bowel movements, and lots of people think we are strange for it, but when something as simple as constipation can cause delirium, you learn to attend well to the simple things.

After my final visit to Roger at home, his son-in-law spoke to me outside the house as I was getting into my car. He told me that Roger's daughter had recently been diagnosed with breast cancer and was undergoing treatment for it. They hadn't told Roger yet, because they did not want to worry him. He wanted my advice about whether this was the right thing to do.

I have never been sure where my authority to advise on such

matters comes from – certainly not from any of the lectures I attended at medical school. However, it is relatively common to be asked to weigh in on family matters of principle, ethics and morality. Usually, I prefer to hesitate to intervene – but not always.

Therefore, I reminded Roger's son-in-law that I had met many people who had come to regret dishonesty but rather fewer who felt the same about the telling the truth. I also suggested that Roger was his sister-in-law's father, and by keeping the news from him, they were denying Roger the chance to be a father and the opportunity to bring to bear his lifetime's experience of joy, loss and love to the situation.

The perspective of older people frequently illuminates how you feel about events, due not just to differences in experiences but also the difference in perspective that longevity brings.

CHAPTER 7

Adapting Healthcare to the Needs of Patients

The healthcare systems that have emerged to meet our needs have failed to keep track of the changing nature of those needs over the last 50 years. The circumstances of older people and those with frailty have been insufficiently accounted for in both the structure and ambition of the health and social care services we currently have in place. Previous chapters have outlined the extent to which ageing and dying have been appropriated by healthcare services, and attention has been drawn to the important aspects of dying that ought to lie outside of healthcare. It should be appreciated that ageing and dying are necessary, perhaps even desirable, but in surrendering the mechanics of ageing to a technological health service, we have at the same time eroded the traditional social structures, such as religion, which gave people meaning and perspective. What has resulted is a modern society in which our capacity to place our individual selves within the timeline of life has been diminished, and instead we find ourselves living in a contemporary world that underlines our individual agency while giving us less perspective for the purpose of our individual experiences as part of a collective.

The success of modern medicine has persuaded us that ageing is a medical problem, and by outsourcing the process of dying to our hospitals and healthcare professionals, we have lost traditional routines of mortality, as well as our familiarity with the sights, sounds and realities of ageing. The expertise for managing the challenges of old age increasingly lies with the field of health and social care and we attend to it late. A de-medicalisation of old age, at least in part, is desirable: only some aspects of old age are amenable to medical intervention. For example, the provision of expert end-of-life symptom control remains an important element of healthcare provision.

The framing of old age and dying within a medical context has some unfortunate consequences. Elisabeth Kübler-Ross[1] points out that death in a hospital is death in a foreign country, where the dying are treated like things. Furthermore, the predominance of medicine in the management of the dying process creates both an unfamiliarity of how we die and uncertainty about when we die:[2] by treating acute illnesses in dying people, we might buy them time but not clemency.

Indeed, by outlining each illness to which an older person succumbs in isolation, we lose the wide angle that allows the overall trajectory to become clear. The tendency of medical practice to deal with discrete episodes of illness leaves doctors poorly prepared to deal with frailty and death. It is only by charting someone's progress over time that one can begin to anticipate their future needs and the likely outcome. The British system of GP-led healthcare should provide the opportunity for this overarching medical view to be taken, but two realities interfere: first, the overwhelming workload of modern GPs means that they have too little time to attend to the needs of their frail and older patients. Second, the decision to send acutely unwell patients to hospital is often made by staff who do not know patients well, outside regular practice hours. In hospital, the knowledge of the patient extends only to the last time they were in hospital. The intervening period is unknown, ensuring that the clinical biography of the patient is described only by their relapses and not their performance and function over the periods in between.

Understanding the potential for medical intervention and appreciating the possible limits for appropriate treatment require an understanding of the life of a patient between episodes of sickness. A frail person in the grip of even a mild infection can look very poorly indeed. What matters is the extent to which they recover and the level at which they function later. Without the context of where a patient has come from, and how they normally function, decisions about medical treatment in hospital are based on the clinical information gathered at the time they present. This is a limited viewpoint: in dealing with older people and those with frailty, the goals for intervention are more nuanced than the information gleaned only from physiological parameters. Supposition and estimates based on first impressions during an acute crisis are no substitute for detailed knowledge and understanding of individual patients built up over time.

Creating an appropriate treatment plan for frail, older patients requires the synthesis of more personal information: what is this person's normal quality of life? What are their own views on the goals for medical intervention? What is their risk-taking style and what are their previously expressed views? These questions are difficult to answer if the team looking after them has never met the patient before.

Frequently, older patients are unable to offer much information due to the prevalence of delirium in acute presentations. Delirium is a state of sudden confusion and poor concentration, often caused by medical problems. Furthermore, the wrong time to be making big decisions about the extent of medical intervention is while in the grip of a crisis. These are questions to be considered carefully, dispassionately, over time and with a good understanding of the person to whom they apply.

The reality of planning care is that it is difficult to articulate in advance all the circumstances with sufficient accuracy that may be encountered in the future. This is the problem with advanced directives – if the specific situation being dealt with is not outlined, they are not valid. Planning care for the frail is not pessimism but rather appreciation that the central question is not if a crisis will occur but when. In fact, one of the hallmarks of frailty is the susceptibility to rapid deterioration in the face of minor physiological insults.[3] Continuity of care over time, through serial crises, allows understanding of the holistic health needs of frail patients: clinical staff appreciate what they are like when they are well, which changes herald a deterioration and even what usually precipitates a crisis. By supporting the patient though the illness, those same team members learn what treatments work and what the typical pattern of recovery is for the individual. It is this type of knowledge that allows medical staff to implement the aspects of care and treatment that make a difference for that person but forego the elements that either make no difference at all or merely subject the patient to excess hazard.

For example, I reviewed a 94-year-old lady at home. A while before, we had looked after her husband in our community hospital in his final days. He had died peacefully and been well cared for. She was grateful for the kindness the staff had shown them both but missed him terribly. She now lived in a care home, where despite her poor vision, crooked spine and deafness, she pottered around the garden, played games with the other residents and listened to her audiobooks. Recently, she had visited her GP complaining of lethargy. Her blood results showed she was anaemic, possibly through the slow loss of blood somewhere along her gut or in her abdomen. She was otherwise OK. In ordinary circumstances, the medical action is simple: the patient is referred to hospital for endoscopies to look at the oesophagus, stomach and duodenum at one end, and the colon at the other end. Neither is very pleasant. I knew this lady from when I cared for her husband. I could see her getting physically frailer but remaining mentally very astute. I knew that much of the meaning of her life had died with her husband, and we could talk openly about her hopes and expectations.

In deciding the right management plan for this lady, we had to consider the risks of the investigations and what we would do with the information gleaned. At her stage of life, the chances of finding a problem about which little can be done, such as a cancer, are high. It is better to consider this before heading down the rabbit hole of investigations. She and I both agreed that endoscopies were too intrusive. I therefore outlined to her that we could manage the anaemia with transfusions and iron replacement but leave the underlying cause unexplored, or we could do a CT scan to look for a cause, with the understanding that it may well reveal a cancer. What I was asking was whether she preferred to know what we were dealing with or whether ignorance was bliss. She chose the former, and we agreed that if the scan showed nothing, apart from managing the anaemia, we would do nothing further. Medical orthodoxy states that a test should only be done if it will change the management plan. She had a scan to look for a problem we would not be able to cure – yet understanding the cause of a problem, even if it is incurable, is useful if it helps the patient come to terms with their own situation and their clinical teams set boundaries and goals for future intervention. She participated fully in the decision-making and was happy with the plan we came up with. She was denied nothing but was spared a great deal of medical intervention.

Such a plan is not impossible in the hospital setting, but it is easier to achieve when the patient has time to consider the options and when they have a therapeutic relationship with their clinicians that has been established over time. The environment is also important: the conversation took place in her home, where she was in charge and I was her guest. That can make a big difference.

It is continuity of care over time and through crises and wellness that creates the circumstances in which the global context of healthcare intervention can be placed. Treating each crisis as a medical problem creates room only for a medical response. Treating each crisis as a medical problem in the context of an individual's personal circumstances gives the space for other factors to come to the fore.

The task at hand is to walk the tightrope between clinical nihilism and optimism. To deny the sick, older patient effective treatment is old-fashioned ageism, but to subject the same person to futile treatment is just as cruel. Finding the most appropriate course for a patient cannot be done based only on their clinical presentation and differential diagnosis. In the absence of context, the decisions about treatment boil down to estimates about the likelihood of cure vs. the risks of side effects and complications. In addition, there is also the requirement for subjective judgements about the quality of life of the person being treated, which in the absence of detailed biographical information is too often fraught with the risks of value judgement.

On the morning of the 7 July 2005, I was sitting in A&E, where I was a Casualty Officer, with my feet up on the desk, trying to decide what to do with a hypothermic, drunk man. I knew nothing about him, except that his temperature was 34.0°C and he was sleeping off a lot of booze. I didn't know his past medical history or if he had a home to go to or money to buy food. Nothing. It's the kind of case that vexes ED doctors because there are so many unknowns – he probably just needed to sober up, but little niggling doubts warn you that these are the patients who become calamitously unwell. I did not know what to do. I was at the start of my first shift after a holiday and had yet to work through my cognitive gears. At that moment, two events saved me – the red emergency phone rang and some people ran into the department from the street, telling us that a tunnel had collapsed at King's Cross. These were the first confusing moments of the aftermath of the 7 July bombings, and the rest of the day was spent tending the wounded. I gave my hypothermic inebriate no further thought until the activity settled down about eight hours later. When I remembered, I asked the charge nurse what had happened to him and was told that he'd been shaken awake and asked to clear the department to make way for the injured. He had walked out and was not seen again.

Knowing so little about this man had made me cautious. Had we not been interrupted, I probably would have admitted him to hospital. For a young man like him, it would have had little long-term impact – it would only have been an overuse of our scarce resources, but I would have reassured myself that it was the safest action to take.

However, for the frail, admission is not a risk-free activity. In fact, it is littered with hazard. Frailty is a condition of diminished physiological reserve, in which minor stressors can lead to profound changes in physical and cognitive function. Any characterisation of hospitals as safe spaces for the frail is misplaced – they are in fact dangerous places. Taken out of their usual environments, hospitals are places of prolonged inactivity, disturbed sleep and changed routine, incubators of infections and environments of heightened falls risk, as well as the places where doctors aggregate and do things to patients.

Any note of flippancy is negated by the starkness of the evidence: brief periods of bed rest can lead to profound loss of muscle strength in older people;[4] the resulting deconditioning leads to an increased risk of falls, delirium, constipation and incontinence.[5] A permanent, functional decline in hospital is experienced by 65% of deconditioned older patients,[6] and this challenges their ability to live independently.

Alongside deconditioning, delirium is one of the other great terrors of those with frailty, causing distressing levels of confusion and agitation. The risk of delirium is highest in patients with dementia and advanced frailty but can be precipitated by pain, disorientation, constipation, urinary catheters, immobility and all manner of medical problems. And while the experience of delirium can be distressing, the outcomes are equally unpalatable: delirium doubles the risk of dying in hospital[7] and confers a higher chance of dying over the next two years.[8]

One would struggle to design an environment better than an acute hospital for exposing the spiralling cycle of complication and despair that affects the ageing human body. The frail patient in hospital may be anchored down by urinary catheters and intravenous (IV) lines, and subjected to a range of tests and treatments, all of which have a complication rate that is disproportionately experienced by the older people. Patients with dementia or delirium, disorientated in time and place, will understandably explore the environment. This is called 'wandering', and while it may be easy to understand from the point of view of a confused patient who does not know where they are or what is happening, to busy ward staff, it is a management problem – their wider responsibilities for numerous patients mean they lack the resources to supervise these patients safely. Instead, 'wandering' is treated as a medical problem and too often managed by the application of antipsychotic medication.

The use of antipsychotics in delirium lacks a strong evidence base.[9] There is some evidence that antipsychotics can help in delirium[10] but there is also evidence that they can worsen outcomes: they can increase the risk of mortality (particularly in those with dementia),[11] as well as increasing the risk of falls and worsening confusion,[12] each of which feeds into separate pathways to poorer outcomes.

Such is the potential web of catastrophe in hospital that it is often true to say that the most effective action a doctor can take to protect the health and well-being of an older person is to discharge them from hospital – or better still, not admit them in the first place.

Thus, the rhetoric about caring for patients in the community is not an absolution of responsibility but recognition that admission to hospital for many older patients heralds an irreversible decline that may well be avoided if the needs of the patient can be met at home. Yet the dangers of hospital admission are too often surrendered to both the desire to cure and the perceived professional risk of not doing everything technically possible. In the common discourse about acute medical care, the failure to recognise and articulate the risks of being in hospital is too often trumped by the expectation that admission to hospital is both safe and the best way to meet the medical needs of the frail.

Here the discussion circles back to the unrealistic expectations we have for the resilience and recovery of the acutely sick and frail. Our failure collectively to attend to the realities of ageing has created a vacuum of preparedness for senescence, while simultaneously creating a medical workforce that is constantly resisting the request to intervene. When the appeals to act are constant and the soul-sapping spectre of complaints is prevalent, it is no wonder that we have developed the tendency to act when wisdom and experience suggest that a more considered approach would be better.

The possibility of caring for frail patients differently is founded on the twin pillars of appropriate decision-making and appropriate systems and services for meeting their needs. Skill is needed to balance the risks. There are times when it is clearly necessary for a patient to go to hospital, regardless of the associated risks, and there are times when it is clearly best avoided, but for all the circumstances in between, the right decision is based on judgement and understanding. Judgement about what the likely outcomes are for the person in front of you; understanding about what the needs of that person are, based on a detailed knowledge of their lives, wishes and goals for intervention.

The ability of any health service to meet the needs of frail patients begins with an understanding of what success looks like. Part of the calculus is the appreciation that in outlining risks, the risks belong to the patient, not to the healthcare professionals involved. Defensive medicine fails on two counts: first, it fails to place the needs of the patient above the needs of the professionals serving their needs. Second, it describes a failure to explore the goals for intervention effectively. Failure to create the opportunity to plan care in advance leaves both patients and doctors unprepared for medical crises, and it is in the empty space where an advance care plan should be that the expectations of patients can depart from that which is possible and doctors begin to worry about how their performance will be appraised by relatives if they fail to apply everything that medicine has to offer.

Done well, advance care plans emerge organically through discussion between clinicians, patients and their families. Often, the substrate for a patient's statement of ambitions rests on a clear description of the medical aspects of their lives and the options available to them. Rarely is it a difficult conversation. Through mutually appreciative conversations, the clinician can start to understand how a patient's health impacts on their quality of daily life, and the patient can begin to understand the nature of the illnesses that restrict them and what the potential and limits for medical intervention are. It is the creation of space for clinical conversations over time that allows for the accommodation of ageing in the clinical management plans for people as they age. Starting such conversations only when people are sick confines the medical care of ageing patients to the realm of the reactive. It is proactive care planning that allows for the right actions to be taken in times of crisis and, as a by-product, creates the opportunity to do less to patients while doing a great deal more for them in the long run.

It is through embedding proactive care planning in routine medical practice for people as they age that we adapt our health services around the needs of the frail, as well as supporting the sustainability of our health services in these straightened times. By outlining the healthcare that is appropriate, we can begin to limit unnecessary activity without unilateral or generalised rationing.

One needn't agree with the premise but dismiss the ambition: how many of you have muttered something along the lines of, 'that's all very well, but it doesn't sound practical/realistic/achievable'? Hope is not a strategy. I am not hoping for change. I know it is possible. How can I say this? My last job was in a healthcare system that is already doing many of the things I describe. We established ways of identifying those with frailty early and planning their care in advance.

We organised community services and our community hospitals around meeting the needs of these patients outside acute hospitals. We learned how to monitor all our admissions and support patients to get home as quickly as possible. We starting tracking patients over time. I stopped doing any clinics and instead saw patients at home; I supported my community colleagues and GPs with the management of their complex patients at home. It wasn't perfect, but in many ways it was brilliant. And we did it without additional funding. Quite simply, we decided it was possible to care for patients with frailty better and we set about trying to do just that. It's a story I would like to share with you, and the next chapter will begin to describe what we did and how we achieved it.

Endnotes

1   Kübler-Ross, E. (1969) *On Death and Dying*. New York: The MacMillan Company.

2   Gawande, A. (2014) *Being Mortal: Illness, Medicine and What Matters in the End*. London: Profile Books.

3   Oliver, D., Foot, C. and Humphries, H. (2014) *Making our Health and Care Systems Fit for an Ageing Population*. London: The King's Fund. Accessed on 10/2/2022 at www.kingsfund.org.uk/sites/default/files/field/field_publication_file/making-health-care-systems-fit-ageing-population-oliver-foot-humphries-mar14.pdf.

4   Tanner, R. E., Brunker, L. B., Agergaard, J., Barrows, K. M. *et al.* (2015) 'Age-related differences in lean mass, protein synthesis and skeletal muscle markers of proteolysis after bed rest and exercise rehabilitation.' *The Journal of Physiology 593*, 18, 4259–4273.

5   British Geriatrics Society (n.d.) *Deconditioning Syndrome Poster*. Accessed on 10/2/2022 at www.bgs.org.uk/sites/default/files/content/attachment/2018-05-03/Deconditioning_syndrome_2_page_poster_0.pdf.

6   British Geriatrics Society (2017) *Deconditioning Awareness*. Accessed on 10/2/2022 at www.bgs.org.uk/resources/deconditioning-awareness.

7   Salluh, J. I. F., Wang, H., Schneider, E. B., Nagaraja, N. *et al.* (2015) 'Outcome of delirium in critically ill patients: Systematic review and meta-analysis.' *British Medical Journal 350*, h2538.

8   Dani, M., Owen, L. H., Jackson, T. A., Rockwood, K., Sampson, E. L. and Davis, D. (2018) 'Delirium, frailty, and mortality: Interactions in a prospective study of hospitalized older people.' *The Journals of Gerontology: Series A, Biological Sciences and Medical Sciences 73*, 3, 415–418.

9   Inouye, S. K., Marcantonio, E. R. and Metzger, E. D. (2014) 'Doing damage in delirium: The hazards of antipsychotic treatment in elderly persons.' *Lancet Psychiatry 1*, 4, 312–315.

10 Neufeld, K. J., Yue, J., Robinson, T. N., Inouye, S. K. and Needham, D. M. (2016) 'Antipsychotic medication for prevention and treatment of delirium in hospitalized adults: A systematic review and meta-analysis.' *Journal of the American Geriatrics Society 64*, 4, 705–714.

11 Maust, D. T., Kim, H. M., Seyfried, L. S., Chiang, C. *et al.* (2015) 'Antipsychotics, other psychotropics, and the risk of death in patients with dementia: Number needed to harm.' *JAMA Psychiatry 72*, 5, 438–445.

12 Inouye, Marcantonio and Metzger (2014).

Harriet

Harriet looked every day of her 94 years. The fatigue of her long years was visible in each wrinkle of her skin, the faintly dusty smell of death that seeped from her pores; it was manifest in the slowness of her movements and the cloudiness of her eyes. It was a terminal tiredness that she felt keenly, understanding too what it meant.

Arrival in hospital often marks the surrender of one's autonomy. Independent of the nature of consultation with staff and the kindness of care, a hospital is a foreign territory of unfamiliar smells and sounds. Hospitals have alienating rhythms that churn along with a momentum of their own. No single person can alter the flow of activity. In a state of distress or suffering, patients arrive in a place where people are always doing something, the meaning of which may be unclear, but with such purpose there seems little point in asking. It is a domain of the new and unfamiliar. It is where suffering and illness take form and are given language. Learning is difficult when one feels unwell, and in hospital there is so much to learn. I have diagnosed cancer hundreds of times, treated thousands of infections and ordered countless tests, and it is the familiarity of these actions that creates the air of competence.

When faced with the unfamiliar, it is usual to look around and see what everyone else is doing. In the absence of cues, it is common to surrender autonomy to the person who seems to know what they are doing. Whether it is right or wrong, that handover of autonomy is usually to the doctor.

'Whatever you say doctor, you are the expert,' is a common answer to my questions. But I am not the expert in being that person.

Harriet was the expert in being Harriet. I had a suspicion of what ailed her, and it would have been easy to send her for the test to diagnose it for certain.

Over the last few months, she had lost her appetite and weight had fallen off her already slender frame, and under the papery skin, one could clearly demarcate her atrophied muscles, overlain with frail blue veins. On her face, the gauntness of impending death had appeared, where the cheek muscles waste away, leaving a hollowness. I could articulate the poor prognostic indicators, but Harriet was living them. I knew she was dying, and in a different language, so did she. It is these conversations that outsiders think must be the hardest, but honesty is only difficult when you are in the habit of lying.

'Harriet,' I said, 'do you have any idea what is wrong with you? Do you want to know what is wrong with you?'

Looking at me boldly, she smiled. 'I don't know what's wrong with me. Do you?'

'I have an idea. The question is whether you want it to have a name. If we go looking for the problem, the chances are that we will find it, but I doubt it is something that I will be able to cure. Once you know what the matter is, there is no way of unknowing.'

'You know best, doctor, I'll go along with what you say.'

'I know the medicine best, but you know yourself better. If I told you that you probably didn't have much time left, would you be surprised?'

Harriet laughed. 'Look at me.' No further qualification was needed, but just in case, she reminded me, 'I'm 94.'

'OK, with that in mind, what is the most important way to spend the time you have left?'

'I want to be at home with my cat.'

'Anything else?'

'Not really.'

'Are you surprised to hear that I think you're dying?'

'No.'

'Do you want to know what you're dying from?'

'I think I'm dying from old age.'

'That's certainly true. But medical practice these days prefers to label the specific illness rather than accept broad statements like that.'

'Would having any tests help you do your job?'

'Not in your case. I know what to do with you.'

'What's that?'

'Get you home to be with your cat and arrange for carers to come in and support you, with the district nurses checking whether you have any symptoms that need treatment.'

'Well let's do that then.'

'And no scan. No buggering about?'

'Sounds perfect.' She lay back on her bed, closed her eyes and smiled.

'You're the boss, Harriet.'

And that's the truth. We work for the benefit of the person in front of us. With the very frail, we often revert them, unbidden, to a child-like state, and we convince ourselves that we know better. Even through the fog of cognitive impairment, deafness, blindness and suffering, no one is better at knowing what it is like to be that older person than that older person. It is not simply a question of autonomy, it is also a matter of expertise. This is often forgotten.

Indeed, it was forgotten by Harriet's daughter, who was in no doubt that her mother had retreated to an infant state. She was also of the class of people who mistake their own professional success for expertise in your domain. She was quick to tell me that she was a barrister. She was quick to tell me that she thought her mother needed a CT scan of her abdomen, and that her friend, who was a top surgeon at a London teaching hospital, agreed.

It is easier to handle someone who thinks you are incompetent after you have spoken to them than someone who makes the same conclusion before they have met you. At least in the former you have had a chance to influence their thinking. In both cases, there is generally an underestimate of the capacity of doctors and nurses to be both insulted and hurt.

She wanted to speak to me away from her mother. It irked her that I sought her mother's permission to do so. When we spoke, I recounted my conversation with her mother.

'Yes, but she wouldn't tell you what she wanted. She's from a different generation.' It's the certainty that always gets me. She rarely saw her mother. She talked with her mother about herself and her children. They hadn't talked about Harriet's health. Harriet's daughter hadn't seen her for a few months and was shocked at her physical deterioration. She wanted to compensate for her absence now by advocating for her effectively. She brought to our meeting the adversarial skills she had honed in the courtroom; the only difference was that we were on the same side.

She came round, eventually, but it took time, and Harriet helped me. Harriet was lucid and steadfast; I kept checking that she was happy with what she had decided. Few decisions are irreversible. Harriet asked her granddaughters to visit her, and the last time I saw her, her daughter, son-in-law and granddaughters were there. There was laughter and Harriet looked contented. She died soon after. She was ready, but her daughter was not. Your career is important, but so is your family.

I have invigilated on hundreds of deaths. Plenty of people wished they had spent more time with their families; not many wished they had spent more time working.

I didn't get her home to be with her cat. No one's perfect.

CHAPTER 8

A Model of Care for Older People

Aspiration is only ever an asymptote: one can tend towards the ideal but never actually reach it. The effort, however, is justified by the outcome – in reaching for the unreachable, we arrive somewhere better than where we set out from. However imperfect it may remain, seeking to improve a health service is always a worthy task.

What matters is that we are trudging up the right hill. Wasted effort is a tragedy of human toil and potential. It is demoralising and disengaging. It creates disconnection between the basic motivation for healthcare staff and the tasks they are set to work on. At its heart, healthcare rests on the simple mantra of doing what the person in front of you needs from you. The perennial trial is marrying the limits of the whole system with the needs of the individual. However, the personalisation of care for frail and older patients should allow limits of intervention to be established and a reasonable platform for practising less medicine on them. That is why the question we keep returning to is what does success look like when we care for our elders? It is a question that is worth considering at leisure, for it is such questions that underline the values that motivate us.

Our ambitions are at risk of being subsumed by the technicalities and demands of an enormous, expensive and pressurised health service. We risk focusing on solutions to the problems without realising that the problems as we see them are the symptoms of deeper-seated issues.

For example, there is evidence that many patients remain in hospital long after their presenting medical issues have been addressed.[1] In the under-nuanced semantics of our time, the patients who are churned through our impenetrable healthcare system are called 'bed-blockers'[2] rather than being more appropriately viewed as the casualties of our system and society – both of which have failed to keep pace with our changing demographics.

Our tendency to treat the processes of delivering healthcare as technical exercises makes us efficient,[3] but it risks also stripping us of our ability to meet the individual needs of the people we serve. To characterise patients as 'bed-blockers', or more recently as 'stranded patients' or 'medically optimised for discharge', is to define their presence in hospital as the problem. It is more aptly understood as a symptom.

Admission to hospital is not a zero-sum game: the arrival or persistence of a patient in hospital does not create capacity elsewhere in the system. It happens either because it is the right action for the patient or because, at the time of presentation, admission to hospital is not only the best option but also the only option. Admission to hospital occurs less through poor individual decision-making and more through the absence of services outside of hospital that could meet the individual's needs. One should resist the notion that there is a simple narrative to explain the issue – a range of factors is involved. The fallout is that older patients are viewed not as a collection of individuals with complex needs but rather as units of activity, for whom the only key target after admission is their discharge.

Somewhere in the matrix of delivering efficient and appropriate healthcare should be the space to deliver care defined by its compassion, kindness and expertise. It is this definition of 'goodness' that is the sustaining motivation for the staff charged with caring. Yet, the amount of effort spent across the health system discussing the qualitative aspects of healthcare delivery is dwarfed by the gigawatts of emotional energy discharged on the issues of 'patient flow' and 'resilience'. It is a telling feature of a tightly controlled system that more time is spent treating the symptoms than correcting the cause.

Let us approach the problem with the maturity of a system that understands its limits, with the participation of people who appreciate that outlining only the problems is destructive. Progress is contingent on the constructive identification of solutions. The emerging thesis is that addressing the needs of those with frailty is founded on understanding their requirements and creating a system that addresses them. Implicit in this synopsis is the assertion that our current system fails to do this.

And yet the system that succeeds where the current one fails can be delivered with the same resources that we have now. It requires transformation but not revolution. Instead, the development of effective frailty services is built on the simple bedrock of clarity of purpose.

Any successful service change requires clear goals. As the saying goes, 'Every system is perfectly designed to get the results it gets.'[4] The development of integrated frailty services in Dorset,[5] for example, was primarily motivated by the desire to provide care for frail patients closer to home to ensure that these patients are only admitted to hospital when their clinical condition requires it and not for the want of services that could meet their needs in the community.

This goal was underpinned by the understanding that patients prefer to be cared for at home[6] but the lack of coordination between community teams meant they often felt overrun by multiple visits from multiple teams.[7] Ten years ago in the NHS, 'integration' was the buzzword. The desire to coordinate services was well meant, but outcomes were muted. Efforts to integrate were undermined by variation in the definition of integration and a failure to appreciate that integration itself is not a goal but rather the means by which a stated goal can be achieved.

Among our community teams in Dorset, we explored the options together and arrived at a version that has a clear vision to manage frailty proactively and responsively, which has defined a function for both community hospitals and community services that is different from other services provided in the area. We defined a niche for community services, which allows us to better meet the expressed needs of our patients while at the same time supporting the pressures across the whole health service. This kind of work is never complete, and I have moved on to another role in a different part of the country, but this work showed me how to define the goal and how to get there. Across the layers of development we implemented, the origins of our work can be stripped right back to a simple, formative process that helped us transform the way we cared for our patients.

Across the health service, one sees examples of rushed implementation: in our haste to implement solutions, we pay too little attention to the details that make the biggest difference. The opening statement of service transformation should focus not on the design of the system you want but on the functioning of the team that will deliver it. The importance of this often-neglected aspect of routine professional function must be emphasised. Highly functional teams are marked out by the presence of shared objectives, interdependence between team members and carving out of time for reflection and review.[8] Furthermore, the creation of teams that operate with high levels of autonomy is associated with improved innovation,[9] performance[10] and patient satisfaction.[11] Autonomous function itself is not an intrinsic function of capable individuals and teams but rather something that flows out of organisations that encourage teams to take time out to reflect and have the habit of celebrating team successes rather than individual triumphs.[12]

For all the magic associated with cultural factors in the workplace, there are very definite actions that lead to the desired professional habits. It is leaders across organisations who create a climate for staff engagement and translate visions into workable objectives.[13]

The role of team leaders is to equip their teams with everything they need to do the job properly – this is a statement not simply of the material items required but also of the process and habits that should be prioritised.

The need for reflective time should not be underestimated. Without setting time aside during the routine schedule for review and open discussion, teams cannot hope to learn from their experiences and innovate accordingly. Learning and innovation occurs when team members have trust in each other, and it is an important leadership action to move from a culture of managing individuals to supporting their teams to monitor and manage the performance of their own team members.[14] Too often the setting aside of time to plan and review work is treated as luxury. It isn't. It is one of the core components of a well-functioning team.

Furthermore, the understanding of what leadership means ought to be tweaked. Successful implementation of a transformation of clinical care requires professional adaptability from the people leading the transformation just as much as it does from the people delivering the care. In the model of leadership described, the function of leadership is to implement a culture of shared objectives, autonomous teams and taking the time to reflect on practice. The goal, therefore, should be the creation of devolved or collective leadership in which the conditions for effective clinical teams are created, allowing them to adapt clinical services around the identified needs of patients. The role of senior management is to support innovation and equip teams with the strategies to succeed.[15] Leadership should be enacted by those with the expertise, capability and capacity to lead,[16] and the individuals both capable and able to lead will vary according to the task.

Creating independence from the direct guidance of organisational leaders is a necessity born out of the need to adapt, respond rapidly and innovate. A dissociation between team members and senior leaders inevitably flows from the separation of senior leaders from direct clinical care. Indeed, a King's Fund survey[17] shows that there is often a discrepancy between the views of the workforce and the executive – the latter often believe in a frontline culture that is not actually real.

The journey to devolved leadership is predicated less on the delivery of process or structure and more on the concern of leaders for others,[18] which means that a key facet of effective leadership is the acknowledgement of the importance of personal fulfilment. It is the central importance of such actualisation that is neglected in the hurly-burly of healthcare operations and management.[19] Through the ten years of the austerity programme, healthcare staff have been exhorted to work faster and harder, ignoring the understanding that this is a workforce capable of very great and sustained effort, best maximised by attending to their needs in the workplace. To surrogate the needs of the staff to the needs of the service is ultimately coun-terproductive: the staff are the service, and creating conditions that diminish their capacity to function at their best (or, indeed, function at all) is self-defeating.

An organisation as large and diverse as the NHS cannot be painted with a single brush. There are of course areas of excellence and enlightened leadership. Yet for those familiar with the NHS, how many of you work within the kind of leadership structure described above? How many of you have met its antithesis? The concept of a true learning organisation is probably a fiction[20] – it is another asymptote. However, it plots the line we should be walking. Strong-arming one's operational ambitions and hopes for a service onto the staff charged with delivering a service is a fast-track route to disengagement. It is not enough simply to deliver one's carefully thought-out plan to staff and expect them to deliver it. Plans con-sidered in isolation from clinical staff will often lack the nuance that frontline experience gives, but more importantly, such plans create the impression that the lived experience of clinicians is unimportant. Collaboration and devolved responsibility are important tools for staff engagement, just as the use of targets and efficiency goals are tools for disengagement.[21] Clinical engagement can be fostered by enacting devolved leadership to clinical teams and allowing time for leadership roles and team development work.[22]

In this indicative overview of the leadership and culture requirements for successful transformation, it should be appreciated that a focus on the softer, qualitative components of the workplace experience is as important as the structures and processes that buttress efficient services. Any sense that carving out the time for reflection or attending to personal fulfilment is indulgent is misplaced: engaged, committed and autonomous teams will set about solving the service delivery issues that can affect any health service. These are the kinds of teams that will understand and discuss the problems and identify the means to solve them with the resources available. These are the kinds of teams that are crucial for the transformation of care around the needs of our patients.

Our own starting point, therefore, was consideration of the existing areas of excellence, the gaps in service provision that prevented us delivering better care and, most importantly, the areas of overlap between the organisational vision and the vision of the individual clinical teams. Our development work found that the absence of personal values from daily work was a strong factor in causing disengagement from service development work. Alignment between the organisational values and individual values was easy to achieve once time was carved out to talk about it.

Indeed, it quickly became apparent that our community teams were brimming with both ideas about how to improve the service and detailed knowledge of the needs and ambitions of our local patients. Successful transformation was therefore quickly established to be dependent on giving flight to the capabilities of the staff who delivered the care, whose capacity for innovation and person-centredness was being stifled by an overly prescriptive and excessively fragmented service. This meant that each health or social care professional who assessed a patient had no access to their colleagues' knowledge about that patient – there were no opportunities to ask, and the record systems were not all aligned.

For example, there were too few opportunities in the regular schedule for community teams to come together to ask for help with their complex patients and to offer their support to colleagues. The result was that each new problem could only be dealt with by referral to another team for assessment. Patients found themselves invaded by multiple teams, and their living rooms became the de facto meeting rooms for community teams.

Frail patients rarely have problems that fit into the neat specialist boxes that we have created. They have needs that transcend the competencies and skills of individual teams. But without a detailed understanding of the patient, finding new problems inevitably leads to more intervention: the more one knows about a patient, the less one tends to actually do. Context is everything in the management of frailty.

Our service transformation did not land fully-formed – successful transformation is always altered by the collision of ambition with real life. We started with conversations about the barriers to excellence and the first steps towards improving the delivery of care. Therefore, our first action was to create regular multidisciplinary team (MDT) meetings for people to discuss their complex cases. The founding basis of these meetings was a simple quid pro quo: access to the expertise of your colleagues is built on each of us returning the favour. Engagement was built upon the utility of the exercise – people attended because it helped them work well, and we discovered that the capacity of all our community health professionals to look after increasingly complex patients at home was enhanced by having easy access to help.

Thus, the starting point was simple: we met once a week to discuss local patients with complex problems. From there, a whole programme developed, based on our learning from each stage of implementation and underpinned by monthly meetings to discuss our work.

In these monthly meetings, the agenda was very simple: we discussed what had worked well, what hadn't worked well and what we wanted to do next. In each MDT and review meeting, there was a purposefully flat hierarchy. The language was informal, and contribution was invited from whoever knew the patient or the problem the best. In a group of mixed professionals, the language that people use to describe the same problem varies – therefore, people need space to describe the issues in their own language and colleagues need the time to ask questions. It doesn't take long, but a particular form of discipline is needed to allow the description or explanation to emerge organically.

I hope this sounds simple. This is what we did. Now, a few years down the line, the service has transformed on many fronts: it has formal processes and systems in place for identifying patients with emerging and worsening frailty and a system for responding to patients experiencing a crisis. It is closely linked with local GPs, and it has a single record system for primary and community services and Health and Social Care Coordinators who monitor and oversee the coordinated work of all the teams. It tracks all of its patients into hospital and supports them back out. It uses its community hospitals as alternatives to acute admission. The changes in my own practice were huge: I didn't do any clinics – instead I saw patients at home and we followed them up as a team.

The growth of our service was organic. There was no way we could have decided in advance how it should look. As we developed confidence and competence, our ability to change and grow emerged. We were guided by the original question of how we could support patients better in their own homes. This was the guiding question, and everything that emerged grew out of our regular discussions about how we could improve the care we delivered to achieve the goal of delivering more care to patients in their own homes.

Endnotes

1   NHS Improvement (no date) *Reducing Long Stays: Where Best Next Campaign.* Accessed on 7/3/2022 at www.england.nhs.uk/urgent-emergency-care/ reducing-length-of-stay/reducing-long-term-stays.

2   Full Fact (2013) *Bed Blocking: What Is It, and Is It Paralysing the NHS?* Accessed on 21/2/2022 at https://fullfact.org/health/bed-blocking-what-it-and-it-paralysing-nhs.

3   Robertson, R. (2017) *How Does the NHS Compare Internationally? Big Election Questions.* London: The King's Fund. Accessed on 10/2/2022 at www.kingsfund.org.uk/ publications/articles/big-election-questions-nhs-international-comparisons.

4   Conway, E. and Batalden, P. (2015) *Like Magic? ('Every System is Perfectly Designed…')* Institute for Healthcare Improvement. Accessed on 10/2/2022 at www.ihi.org/ communities/blogs/origin-of-every-system-is-perfectly-designed-quote.

5   Dorset Healthcare (2016) *New Care 'Hub' Transforms Services for People in Weymouth and Portland.* Accessed on 7/3/2022 at https://www.dorsethealthcare.nhs.uk/ about-us/news-events/press/new-care-hub-transforms-services-people-weymouth-and-portland.

6   Social Care Institute for Excellence (2014) *What Older People Want: Commissioning Home Care for Older People.* Accessed on 10/2/2022 at www.scie.org.uk/ publications/guides/guide54/what-older-people-want.asp.

7   Dharamshi, R. (2014) 'The future of care for frail elderly patients: Our first steps towards progress.' *Postgraduate Medical Journal 90,* 1066, 427–428.

8   West, M., Alimo-Metcalfe, B., Dawson, J., El Ansari, W. *et al.* (2012) *Effectiveness of Multi-Professional Team Working (MPTW) in Mental Health Care. Final Report.* London: NIHR Service Delivery and Organisation Programme.

9   West, M. and Anderson, N. (1996) 'Innovation in health care teams.' *Journal of Applied Psychology 81,* 6, 680–693.

10 Macy, B. and Izumi, H. (1993) 'Organizational Change, Design and Work Innovation: A Meta-Analysis of 131 North American Field Studies – 1961–1991.' In W. Pasmore and R. Woodman (eds), *Research in Organizational Change and Development* (pp.235–313). Greenwich, CT: JAI.

11 Borrill, C., West, M., Carter, M. and Dawson, J. (2004) *The Relationship Between Staff Satisfaction and Patient Satisfaction.* Accessed on 10/2/2022 at https://www. affinaod.com/wp-content/uploads/2015/01/Staff-Satisfaction-and-Patient-Satisfaction.pdf.

12 *Ibid.*

13 West, M., Eckert, R., Steward, K. and Pasmore, B. (2014) *Developing Collective Leadership for Health Care.* London: The King's Fund. Accessed on 10/2/2022 at www. kingsfund.org.uk/publications/developing-collective-leadership-health-care.

14 West, M. and Borril, C. (2005) 'The Influence of Team Working.' In J. Cox, J. King, A. Hutchinson and P. McAvoy (eds), *Understanding Doctors' Performance* (pp.106–122). Oxford: Radcliffe.

15 West and Anderson (1996).

16 *Ibid.*

17 The King's Fund (2014) *Culture and Leadership in the NHS: The King's Fund 2014 Survey*. London: The King's Fund. Accessed on 10/2/2022 at www.kingsfund. org.uk/publications/culture-and-leadership-nhs.

18 Alimo-Metcalfe, B. and Alban-Metcalfe, J. (2005) 'Leadership: Time for a new direction.' *Leadership 1*, 51–71.

19 Riley, W., Davis, S. E., Miller, K. K. and McCullough, M. (2010) 'A model for developing high-reliability teams.' *Journal of Nursing Management 18*, 5, 556–563.

20 Branson, C. M. (2008) 'Achieving organisational change through values alignment.' *Journal of Educational Administration 46*, 3, 376–395.

21 The King's Fund (2013) *Patient-Centred Leadership. Rediscovering our Purpose*. London: The King's Fund. Accessed on 10/2/2022 at www.kingsfund.org.uk/ sites/default/files/field/field_publication_file/patient-centred-leadership-rediscovering-our-purpose-may13.pdf.

22 Maben, J., Peccei, R., Adams, M., Robert, G. *et al.* (2012) *Exploring the Relationship Between Patients' Experience of Care and the Influence of Staff Motivation, Affect and Wellbeing*. London: National Institute for Health Research Service Delivery and Organisation Programme.

Deirdre

Deirdre had a problem: she needed help at home. She had struggled for two years after her husband died, but theirs was an old-fashioned marriage, in which he earned the wage, paid the bills and fixed anything that was broken, while she looked after the cooking, the cleaning and the children. When he retired from his job as a plumber, he took responsibility for the garden, the allotment and the household chores, which she found increasingly difficult to manage. At the end of each month, they would sit down together and balance the cheque book. It was a division of labour that worked for them for the 58 years they were married. Following his death, she grieved in the way that many of her generation grieve – privately, while pretending to everyone else that she was OK.

Yet, she could never keep on top of the housework, the laundry and the cooking. Her children suspected she was finding it difficult, but she was too embarrassed to let them visit. She would find an excuse to cancel their visits, or when they came over to take her out, she would always be waiting for them outside her front door.

While she was able to keep them from seeing the mounting squalor at home, she was less able to maintain her appearance. She started to lose weight, her clothes were dirty and she started to smell. She was proud, so her children didn't mention it. They put blankets on the sofa whenever she visited.

Eventually, Deirdre was admitted to hospital, when her neighbour noticed that she had not been seen for a few days. They called the police, who broke through her door and found her lying on her sofa – soiled and septic from a urine infection caused by her becoming so constipated she was unable to empty her bladder.

In hospital, Deirdre initially pretended that she could manage by herself, but the occupational therapist was gently persistent and she eventually relented and allowed her to visit her home. The occupational therapist was not surprised by what she found. Deirdre's story is disappointingly common.

The real kicker, however, is that one only qualifies for state-funded social care when one has less than £23,250 in savings. Until that point, an individual is responsible for all the costs of their care, unless they can demonstrate exceptional or complex needs (Deirdre's were not).

The cliff edge of means testing of social care is particularly brutal for Deirdre and her generation. Many of them worked hard, thriftily putting a little aside each month, year after year, hoping to be able to leave something to their children.

One day, I visited Deirdre on the ward and found her holding a quotation for her planned care package. It was set to cost her £1200 a month. She had £50,000 in her savings account. She was heartbroken to be cheating her children of their inheritance.

The next week, she returned home with her package of care. The following week, she cancelled it, as was her right. A month later, she was found on the floor with a broken hip. She was admitted to hospital, where she had an emergency fixation of the fracture. However, in her weakened state, she found it difficult to walk after the operation and developed a pneumonia. Two weeks after the operation, she was dead.

CHAPTER 9

Effective Teams

The need, in the previous chapter, to emphasise the importance of team dynamics in service development is both necessary and slightly embarrassing. It should be self-evident that good staff engagement is a basic requirement for successful change management, but experience suggests that in our prolonged time of strain, it is forgotten. Effective team functioning is itself a worthy ambition with its own intrinsic value; it is also part of the solution to several problems experienced across the NHS.

Highly functioning teams by themselves, however, are insufficient to guarantee effective services. The manner of service developments sits alongside team development as an important facet of improving services. A positive notion of service development exists, not only as a reaction to how change is managed in practice, but also as an affirmative statement of how change should be managed. There are a few home truths about change management and service improvement in the NHS in general, and frailty services in particular, that have to be acknowledged before they can be addressed.

For example, it should be appreciated that regardless of its nature, change is associated with chaos and loss.[1] Thus, in the disruptive environment of change in the workplace, clinical engagement is contingent on clinical ownership of both the problems and the solutions. Chaos is more tolerable when it is one's own.

In viewing the current state of clinical services, it is apparent that the structure of older person care services focuses too much on the provision of acute care[2] and that the shape of health services is significantly influenced by the supply-side dynamics of the health service[3] – the nature of care received by the patients tends to be determined by the structures and limitations of the service rather than their needs.

Data is widely used in the appraisal of the performance of health services, but often without enough discipline. Repeatedly, figures are used as the basis on which to draw conclusions about the development need, but as Don Berwick has pointed out,[4] metrics can highlight problems and direct inquiry, but 'culture will trump rules, standards and control strategies every time'. Numbers tell their own type of story, but the successful use of data involves looking for the problems in the areas they point to and then creating a narrative that fits with the human element of the story.

For example, a team is less likely to respond to the news that their length of stay is too long than they are to the appreciation that aspects of their internal processes could help them improve patient care. To focus only on solving length of stay is to ignore the multitude of human factors that underpin sustainable and acceptable solutions. For example, we started to use 'red' and 'green' days to highlight the progress of our patient: a green day is a day when something designed to help a patient's progress is taking place, while a red day is one on which nothing meaningful is happening. The ideal patient experience is for a series of green days, at the end of which they go home. Outlining our own work in terms of how useful the day is for the patient is more meaningful to me than simply saying the length of stay is too long. I am minded to apologise to no one if a patient has a long length of stay of green days.

What the observation above alludes to is the understanding that in the absence of clinically meaningful narratives, targets and efficiency goals are a barrier to clinical engagement.[5] Furthermore, the most effective change is enacted by organisations motivated by values,[6] meaning that clinical metrics by themselves lack both nuance and persuasive powers in practice.

The advantage of values-based practice is that it creates the space to align the design of services with patient-based outcomes: it is only possible to understand what high-quality care is by asking patients, and it is only by listening to patients that one can develop a culture in which patients come first.[7]

Thus, sitting alongside the important consideration of how teams function is the important consideration of how they are motivated to develop their services. Values alignment and patient-centred care all derive from organisational values and habits, which must be embedded at all levels: a values-driven, patient-centred team will be suffocated in an organisation that does not share the same value set or allow for its expression.

Therefore, while there is a pressing need for NHS organisations to instil in their teams the confidence for clinical self-expression, it is equally important that the ambitions of the clinical staff relate closely to the higher-level ambitions of senior management. Often, this is expressed as a function of the dialogue from 'ward to board', but in fact, the risk of Chinese whispers as a message passes either up or down an organisation should be mitigated by all levels of the organisation deriving their approach from the same primary source – the patient.

Patient-centred care always runs the risk of becoming a platitude, and indeed, in designing services for older people and those with frailty, there is the hazard of being misled through engaging with the wrong types of service user. There are six stated principles of patient-centred care, ranging from coordination and integration to equality and third-sector involvement. It is frustratingly tautological that the first principle listed on the Health Education England web-site[8] states that person-centred care is 'person-centred: personalised, coordinated and empowering'. Armed with that description, who could fail to be both inspired and informed.

Services ought to be aligned to the perceived and expressed needs of their patients, yet it is less clear what this involves in practice. There is a lot of talking about aligning services to patients, and, typically, organisations will talk to local patient groups when embarking on service redesign. Yet these tend to be self-selecting groups, who are both willing and able to participate. In frailty, many service users are unable to participate (after all, they are frail) and unwilling: they are not used to being heard, and the expression of honest views is tempered by the fear that it will negatively influence the care they are given.

Better, perhaps, than designing a service around the outcomes of distinct patient engagement events is to instil individual responsiveness and adaptability in the daily routine of clinical services. Truly patient-centred care is contingent on responding to the needs of the person in front of you rather than applying the model of care developed from patient engagement to the person in front of you. What matters is that the services have the scope to be flexible. Effective frailty services are probably built on having the capacity and the capability to respond directly to the ambitions and needs of each frail person differently.

One has to say 'probably', as while there is a great deal of evidence about what doesn't work, there is rather less about what does work.[9] Rossi[10] summarises that the failure of innovations to demonstrate impact can be attributed to a poor understanding of the underlying cause of the problem, poor design of programmes to address a correctly identified cause and poor implementation of an appropriate intervention. Failures at all three levels abound across the NHS. Yet, the greatest confounder to embedding the principles of good frailty care in routine practice are the overbearing demands of 'now', which prevent us ever fully attending to the needs of the future. It is trolley waits in EDs and lack of beds in acute hospitals that command the attention both of mainstream media and health service management. It is to these areas that resources are hoovered at times of strain, but this is only ever crisis management, or palliation – it is not a solution to the underlying problems.

Meeting the true needs of frail patients asks us to take attention away from the areas where pressure is being felt the most. High demand on EDs is solved by solutions outside of ED. It is always appropriate to embed systems that deal well with older patients in acute hospitals, but such systems won't address the root causes. This is more than a demand-management problem – it is a needs-management problem, in which the needs of our prevalent patients are being dealt with by a system designed to address a different set of requirements. One argument that I am trying to weave through this book is that success is built on having a clear understanding of what success looks like and then building a system to meet that need. Heroic exertions are praiseworthy, but they are no basis for lasting achievement.

For the purpose of this chapter, the equation that must be balanced is the capacity of a health system that is routinely bursting its banks, with the individual needs of a growing cohort of patients with frailty who are significant users of our flooded health service.

One central component of the thesis about frailty services through this book is the appreciation that, in the context of the inevitable but variably expressed vagaries of ageing, there are circumstances in which patients should be offered and given the whole gamut of medical and surgical interventions; but, equally, there are times when they should not. Limits should be placed on intervention through the marriage of understanding the balance of risk vs. benefit, and futility vs. cure, with the understanding of what the patient wishes to achieve.

The point is that ageing, as with life, is probably not ontological (we do not fit into neat categories), but in fact more phenomenological (personal experience is reality). Thus, however hard and high modern medicine reaches for the empirical and the objective, there will often be a disconnect between the views of the medical practitioners and the patients they serve. For example, patient-centred care is undermined by the dominance of a biomedical model in healthcare,[11] and during times of strain, staff tend to revert to a disease-centred model of care.[12] The truth is that the decision-making of health professionals and patients is often underpinned by different basic philosophies.

Squaring this circle will always be an approximation, yet great strides can be taken from the very simple starting point of the practitioner asking the question, 'What does success look like?' It is this question that frames medical intervention in the form of the personal, the biographical and even the phenomenological; it allows for appropriate filaments of medical empiricism to buttress the lives of the patients it serves but not dominate or overpower them.

The landscape for the proposed style of advanced decision-making is outside of the acute crisis. During a crisis, decision-making is skewed by the call for urgency in the context of bilateral unfamiliarity: the medical team does not know the patient and the patient knows neither the people caring for them nor the situation in which they find themselves.

My own frailty services began with the development of rapid response services for local patients, but we quickly realised that the sooner we learned about emerging problems, the easier it was to enact a response other than referral to acute hospital. This has an obvious logical end point: frail people will inevitably hit a crisis. Therefore, it cannot be too early to prepare.

Thus, two parallel work streams have emerged: proactive and reactive pathways, and it is the development of the proactive pathways that has unlocked the potential of our service. The reactive response (i.e. what we do when a crisis starts) is bolstered by the prep work that has already taken place around the patient and consists of the coordination of local community services and the request that people referring in to the service do their best to describe the problem, so that we can figure out what can be done with the resources available. In the past, referrers were expected to identify the problem, diagnose the solution and then find the correct team to implement it. This was a frustrating and time-consuming experience of ringing the wrong team, or the right team with no capacity to help, and ended up with the patient being referred to hospital.

The proactive work consists of the community teams taking part in the regular frailty meetings at local GP practices to discuss patients with emerging or worsening frailty, planning assessments and multidisciplinary input, reviewing the patients who have been admitted to hospital since the last meeting and using tools such as the eFI (electronic Frailty Index) to check if we know who the frail patients are.

None of this immediately impacts on the patients turning up to ED or the Acute Medical Unit, but delivered consistently over time, the benefits begin to tell. In Dorset, the areas with the most mature integrated community hubs have experienced falling levels of emergency admissions for their local older patients and those patients spend less time in hospital. But that is not the whole of it, indeed, it is probably not even the most important part of it. There may be overlap between services that care well for older patients with frailty and services that support the pressures on the acute hospital, but they are not the same.

Instead, the system proposed for older people is one in which the aims for medical intervention are framed in terms of the ambitions of the patient. This benefits the patient, it benefits the staff who deliver the care and it benefits the whole system by personalising care, improving the experience of staff delivering care and limiting the application of futile interventions. Indeed, it is the qualitative aspects of our service development that are the most compelling: staff satisfaction rates have risen, patient experience has improved and we have developed a fruitful, rewarding partnership with our local GPs. It is these aspects of our own programme that make it feel like the right work to be doing, as well as making our service changes feel sustainable. They have been designed by the staff who deliver them and fit with the values that motivate them.

The trap that we fall into repeatedly in the NHS is measuring what we can count. Whenever I presented the work that we had done in Dorset, and outlined the importance of personalisation, enacting a strong value set in service development and focusing on team performance, I was always asked, 'Yes, but what has been the impact on acute hospitals?' It is easy to count how many patients have been admitted to hospital and how long they spent there. It is hard to capture the qualitative aspects of patient care that make the most difference to the patients themselves – yet for older people, this is where our attention really should be.

Endnotes

1   Elrod, P. D. and Tippett, D. D. (2002) 'The "death valley" of change.' *Journal of Organizational Change Management 15*, 3, 273–291.

2   Cornwell, J. (2012) *The Care of Frail Older People with Complex Needs: Time for a Revolution.* London: The King's Fund. Accessed on 15/2/2022 at www.kingsfund. org.uk/sites/files/kf/field/field_publication_file/the-care-of-frail-older-people-with-complex-needs-mar-2012.pdf.

3   The Health Foundation (2014) *Helping Measure Person-Centred Care.* London: The Health Foundation. Accessed on 15/2/2022 at www.health.org.uk/publications/ helping-measure-person-centred-care.

4   Berwick, D. (2012) Improving the Safety of Patients in England. Accessed on 15/2/2022 at www.kingsfund.org.uk/audio-video/don-berwick-improving-safety-patients-england-presentation-slides.

5   The King's Fund (2013) *Patient-Centred Leadership: Rediscovering our Purpose.* London: The King's Fund. Accessed on 15/2/2022 at www.kingsfund.org.uk/ sites/files/kf/field/field_publication_file/patient-centred-leadership-rediscov-ering-our-purpose-may13.pdf.

6   Branson, C. M. (2008) 'Achieving organisational change through values alignment.' *Journal of Educational Administration 46*, 3, 376–395.

7   The King's Fund (2013).

8   Health Education England (n.d.) *Person-Centred Care.* London: HEE. Accessed on 15/2/2022 at www.hee.nhs.uk/our-work/person-centred-care.

9   Edwards, N. (2014) *Community Services: How They Can Transform Care.* London: The King's Fund. Accessed on 15/2/2022 at www.kingsfund.org.uk/sites/default/ files/field/field_publication_file/community-services-nigel-edwards-feb14.pdf.

10 Rossi, P. H., Lipsey, M. W. and Freeman, H. E. (2004) *Evaluation: A Systematic Approach*, 7th ed. Thousand Oaks, CA: Sage.

11 Pelzang, R. (2010) 'Time to learn: Understanding patient-centred care.' *British Journal of Nursing 19*, 14, 912–917.

12 Ekman, I., Swedberg, K., Taft, C., Lindseth, A. *et al.* (2011) 'Person-centered care: Ready for prime-time.' *European Journal of Cardiovascular Nursing 10*, 248–251.

Katie and Rebecca

When COVID-19 landed on my ward at the end of March 2020, it seemed to waft through like a phantom. Each time you turned around, a positive test came back in someone new – often without symptoms. Our first patient to come back positive was someone who didn't really fit the criteria for testing, but we elected to do it on him anyway, so that when the crisis hit properly, we would be slicker at the convoluted process of taking and processing the swabs.

With each positive test, it became impossible not to internally tot up the number of times you had seen that patient without protective equipment. Healthcare professionals reacted to the looming arrival of COVID-19 the same way that everyone does. They are, after all, normal people. Some were concerned for their own welfare, others for their families and also for the patients. Some were very relaxed about the whole affair. Overall, the tension, however, was tangible. Healthcare staff are good at dealing with the emergencies they have prepared for, trained for or previously experienced. This, however, was all new and unpredictable.

I balk slightly at the characterisation of healthcare staff as heroes. It creates the impression that they are capable of, and expected to deliver, the impossible. Being a hero implies an element of sacrifice. We should not expect this of our NHS staff, and their willingness to take risks is not an absolution of the requirement to provide basic and available protection.

Some of my colleagues with underlying health problems were told to isolate themselves at home. Their emotions ranged from relief to frustration and even embarrassment. Other staff ploughed on, day after day, shift after shift, as their colleagues succumbed and had to remain at home.

What sticks in my mind, however, is the memory of a nurse and a healthcare assistant, Katie and Rebecca, on the first weekend it all started. As I walked past them, they were helping each other don their protective equipment before entering a side room to wash a patient. From inside the room, I could hear them chatting and joking with him as they helped him with his daily ablutions. It was a moment of two people doing their normal job in abnormal circumstances. There was nothing heroic about what they did, but it was a reminder that many jobs are worth doing, and worth doing well. When circumstances make that job more difficult, all you can do is your best.

For a while, at the start of the pandemic, we applauded these staff on our doorsteps. Yet Katie and Rebecca carry out this kind of work, week after week, without recognition (and without a pay rise for ten years).

Chapter 10

Public Service Motivation

Medicine can be a tricky life. There is often the nagging sense that that the job is trying to hurt you. Low points come and go, when we wonder if we're good enough, kind enough, robust enough. I've ruminated on my mistakes, my unkindnesses and my personal failings. I am often sustained by the realisation that being my best possible version of a doctor is a good use of my time.

However, the winds of change are blowing. I sense a general trend of jadedness and ennui from those around me. There is the perpetual suspicion that we are not valued: we know that we value each other, and that some of our patients value us, but we wonder if wider society really does.

I recently discovered that tax rules meant I would soon be paying to continue in the leadership role I had taken on – paying to do a job that on occasions had left me with a tiredness that no amount of sleep could fix, a job that found me sometimes sitting on the edge of the bed on dark mornings searching for the energy to start the day, a job that occupied my mind, distorted my home life and robbed me of relaxation. That was when I realised I was making the transition from public servant to patsy.

We often talk about whether the NHS is well enough funded, but no amount of money can provide the staff to do the work if the right staff either do not exist or do not want to work for the NHS. For too long we have ignored the need to look after the people who deliver the care. The creation of a sustainable workforce is the biggest issue we need to address. It bothers me that healthcare professionals are expected to continue to work under ever more strenuous situations with little sign that they are appreciated. The nature of healthcare work means that it will always be emotionally and physically demanding. Yet we compound the intrinsic pressures of the work with the way we organise, underfund and squeeze staff. Are we all patsies? Are healthcare staff motivated by the desire to care being exploited to prop up an understaffed and under-resourced health service?

If you ask junior doctors and medical students what motivates them, they will tell you that medicine is defined by 'responsibility to others', which they define as requiring altruism.[1] Doctors seem to enjoy medicine for the benefit to patients, for the technical and scientific component of their work and to satisfy their intellectual curiosity.[2] Some feel that altruism should be a prerequisite for a career in medicine,[3] but this rather depends on how one defines altruism. There is perhaps a traditional view of doctors as selfless,[4] and there is still a compassionate value set that defines medical practice: the General Medical Council's *Good Medical Practice* states that, 'good doctors make patients their first concern,'[5] and 'integrity, trustworthiness and compassion' are still stated ideals for doctors,[6] but it is not clear that altruism really is a desirable attribute for modern doctors.

There is considerable overlap between concepts such as altruism, public service motivation and prosocial motivation. What distinguishes altruism from other social behaviours is a person's action to create a benefit for someone else at the expense of themselves: altruism involves at least a degree of personal cost and is more correctly understood as a behaviour rather than a motivation.[7] The underlying motivation for altruists is less relevant, therefore, than the outcome that results.

A behavioural definition of altruism takes me back to the days of my psychology degree. I don't know the current academic biases of this field, but in the early 2000s it was all about cognitive psychology, which consisted, as far as I could work out, of a series of flow diagrams illustrating the cognitive processes that took place in our minds. What irked me about it was the pointlessness of all the speculation of these elaborate flow diagrams mapping out brain processes entirely divorced from neuroscience. It was a like a modern-day version of the Reformation debates about transubstantiation: lots of brain power devoted to an illusion of human construction.

The antithesis of cognitive psychology at that time was behavioural psychology. It was deeply unfashionable. Yet it was honest and often compelling. It is based on the appreciation that in explaining human (or animal) behaviour, we can see and control inputs, and we can observe and record outputs. We cannot fathom what goes on in the brain, and it is pointless to guess. Understanding behaviour can be usefully advanced by carefully correlating inputs and outputs, and choosing the most parsimonious (i.e. simplest) relationship between the two.

Such an approach can be an apt way of understanding the behaviours of healthcare staff: there are a range of motivations for the caring professions, and one gains little from cataloguing them individually or into themes. However, one learns a great deal from understanding how caring behaviours are influenced by the environment they work in.

It surprises no one, except economists, that healthcare staff are motivated by factors other than money. In fact, there is plenty of evidence to suggest that financial rewards can even dislodge people from their non-financial motivation, resulting in less caring activity.

Thus, we enter the realm of intrinsic motivation, which can be described as the motivation, 'to perform an activity when one receives no apparent reward except the activity itself'.[8] In an age dominated by neoliberal economics, it baffles economists to learn that money is not the only motivator and can even demotivate.[9] Intrinsic motivation is largely ignored by mainstream economics, revealing the neoliberal lie we have tied ourselves up with: when Margaret Thatcher declared that, 'there is no such thing as society,' she was both wrong and channelling the neoliberal economist Friedrich August von Hayek.[10] At the risk of reductionism, the neoliberal view can be summarised as the view that all utility has a monetary price, and this value will be determined by the free market. Failure to achieve a price is either a function of constrained markets or an absence of utility. This is the attitude that underpins the modern obsession with 'monetising' resources such as woodlands or open spaces. The influence of neoliberal economics is something we can review at leisure, while considering the success of mainstream economics to reduce human behaviour to the action of individuals as economic agents. It is not just our gullibility we need to review, but also the persuasion of the neoliberal promise of economic growth, as defined by gross domestic product (GDP), being a national ambition worth sacrificing other, non-monetary benefits for.

The lie is revealed, at least in part, by the behaviour of real people, as opposed to the economic automatons that economists imagine us to be. Titmuss[11] showed that introducing payments for blood donations reduces blood donations and proposed that the introduction of money undermines the idea of social obligation, which encourages us to do something socially beneficial. Paying for it turns it into a service rather than a public good. Perhaps more profoundly, Frey and Jegen[12] describe a Swiss survey which revealed that when financial incentives were introduced as a means of garnering support for the siting of a nuclear waste facility, half the number of local people supported the proposals than when no money at all was involved.

This 'crowding out' of intrinsic motivation by financial rewards is proposed to act through a number of mechanisms, from incentives increasing the perceived pressure and causing 'choking'[13] to external motivators reducing feelings of self-determination;[14] those who maintain intrinsic motivation in the face of financial incentives feel 'over-justified' and therefore reduce the elements of motivation under their control. Introducing money turns any action into a transaction and invites value judgements. When considered in terms of money, therefore, many intrinsically motivated people realise that they too are patsies and withdraw their labour and commitment.

Offering financial incentives can imply that the individual competence and motivation that previously drove performance is unimportant and not appreciated. The offer of rewards for performance undermines self-regulation and results in people taking less responsibility for themselves.[15]

Regulating strongly crowds out intrinsic motivation and is counterproductive. A similar effect is seen in healthcare, where performance metrics have been used to drive performance – even though this doesn't work.[16] Performance data creates the aura of accountability and governance but does not actually improve performance. Instead it undermines trust between clinicians and managers by shifting the locus of the interactions from interpersonal relationships between them to what the numbers show.

The scenarios outlined have been elegantly described by Julian Le Grand,[17] who identifies knights (public-spirited altruists) and knaves (self-interested people). The introduction of financial incentives turned knights into knaves. He observes that knights can be 'act relevant' (the act leads to the gratification) or 'act irrelevant' (the gratification results from the person needing help getting help, regardless of who delivers it). This harks back to the hidden motivations I talked about earlier, and the key being the behaviour that results rather than the underlying thought processes.

For example, the intrinsic motivation of doctors may mean that they are driven less by their concerns for individual patients and more by their ambition to deliver a good service. Indeed, one might consider healthcare professionals motivated by service-level ambitions to be more desirable than those driven by self-sacrificing altruism. The utility of an equitable health service involves balancing the needs of the person in front of you with the wider needs of the whole population. Furthermore, we should want our healthcare professionals to have sustainable and enjoyable careers rather than watch them burn themselves out at the sharp end of their altruism.

Perhaps, therefore, we should be seeking ways to channel the intrinsic motivation of our healthcare professionals, while at the same time making it clear that a good doctor or nurse is not someone who burns themselves out but rather seeks to create a system of healthcare that allows patients to experience good care from staff who are enabled to be the best healthcare professional they can be.

The current healthcare system, and indeed society, considers the thinking of the previous paragraph to be fanciful.

In researching this chapter, I have come across papers, which, after describing the crowding out of intrinsic motivation by financial rewards, have concluded that the effective running of public services requires the low pay of staff so that only people with strong intrinsic motivation are attracted to the roles.[18] One has to wonder about the intrinsic motivation of someone who recommends, 'Treat 'em mean and keep 'em keen' as public policy. One must also be careful of conflating 'value' with 'motivation'.

It says something of the power of intrinsic motivation that relatively low paid professions, such as nursing, remain popular – but low pay is not required to preserve intrinsic motivation. It is perfectly appropriate to pay nurses a good wage – indeed, they would probably appreciate it. What matters is the creation of working cultures and environments that allow for caring behaviours. The underlying motivation is not important – it is the behaviours that matter: that the roles that staff take on give them the time and space to act with compassion. It is relentlessness, pressure, stress and unhappiness that stifle kindness. Predicating pay rise on performance gains won't work, as it devalues the commitment already shown.

Within healthcare management, there is a frequent failure to appreciate that most healthcare staff do not need to be motivated – what they need is for their intrinsic motivation (the motivation that sustained them through years of training, the motivation that has sustained them through the last ten years) to be given room to blossom.

We spend so long in the NHS gripping performance so tightly and squeezing every last ounce of productivity out of people that we do not stop to question why it is so hard. It needn't be hard, and it wouldn't be if we realised that the secret to getting the most from staff is to support them to be the living embodiment of whatever their intrinsic motivation is and let their professional autonomy flourish. We need to mature from 'managing people' to creating and supporting teams. A good manager identifies the needs and capabilities of their team members and supports and coaches them to success.

I am not talking about a workplace free-for-all, where people choose what to do and what not to do. Instead, I am telling you that micro-managing doesn't work in healthcare and that for the intrinsically motivated, a different form of management is needed.

An effective management strategy focuses on providing teams with the resources needed to do the job properly, a clear understanding of what success looks like (aligned to their own values) and regular information telling them how they are doing. Teams should be managed as teams, not as collections of individuals – successes are shared by the group and failures are used as collective learning opportunities. Innovation is encouraged, autonomy allowed and failures expected. Managers are there to help, to coach and to keep the team functioning as a unit.

A team managed in this way will give you the best it is capable of, but it may not give you everything you want or need. The problem comes when, as in the NHS, you want it to deliver more than it is reasonably resourced for.

I know how staff in the NHS respond to crises of the very gravest kind. I saw it on 7 July 2005, when I was working in A&E at University

College Hospital in London; I am seeing it right now in the coronavirus pandemic. The NHS sparkles with shining examples of humanity, with sacrifice ranging from the routine to the extraordinary. The staff of the NHS are capable of stepping up to any emergency, but not endlessly – and this is the problem: the last 12 years have been a slow-burn crisis of demand never-endingly outstripping resources. The effort has been valiant, but it cannot last forever.

The demotivation of healthcare staff has not emerged from the inappropriate use of financial incentives but instead from the possibly cynical over-reliance on their intrinsic motivation to compensate for insufficiencies in cash and staff. There is an important but often missed distinction between creating optimum conditions for team and individual performance and maximising the offer of discretionary efforts.

Working beyond the requirements of one's formal job role should only ever be an individual choice – it should never form part of work plans to increase discretionary effort. As soon as one starts to rely on the offer of discretionary effort, it becomes unpaid labour. Bolino and friends[19] call discretionary work 'organisational citizenship behaviour' (OCB) and note that it may arise from, 'positive job attitudes, positive affect, encouraging leadership and a supportive organisational climate'. These are all positive factors to be encouraged and appreciated in the workplace, but there is also danger in the absence of sufficient organisational discipline: in organisations where displays of OCBs are common, they may be so prevalent that they are expected. People may engage in OCBs as a distraction from their boring work role or to demonstrate their value to the organisation in a self-serving way. Importantly, when sustained over time, OCBs may come to be considered part of the core work role and no longer optional.[20]

In this latter scenario, the expectation to deliver discretionary effort contributes to 'stress and overload',[21] as well as higher levels of conflict between work and family and leisure, and intention to quit.[22] When discretionary effort goes unrecognised, counterproductive work behaviours may result[23] and the core work role may be neglected.

Non-financial factors can crowd out intrinsic motivation – the literature tells us that constraining autonomy can reduce the intrinsic motivation of staff.[24] Common sense tells me also that if we routinely exploit staff, by expecting them to do ever more with ever less, even the most altruistic staff will either choose to leave or break themselves trying to keep up. The literature also tells us that intrinsic motivation can be crowded in through the promotion of professional development, giving staff the opportunity to take part in research or teaching and recognising their achievements, merit awards and allowing them to develop their services. What this speaks about is the idea that good leadership and management in the NHS, at least, is characterised by having concern for the staff you work with. Taking the time to understand the needs, concerns and ambitions of your team members will allow them to flourish and find reward in the work they do. It is not about squeezing performance out of people or tricking them into giving more than they are paid for. Good leadership is defined simply by the boundaried ambition to help your team members flourish, in whatever individual way that they can.

Endnotes

1   Chard, D., Elsharkawy, A. and Newbery, N. (2006) 'Medical professionalism: The trainees' views.' *Clinical Medicine 6*, 1, 68–71.

2   Chard, Elsharkawy and Newbery (2006).

3   Harris, J. (2017) 'Altruism: Should it be included as an attribute of medical professionalism?' *Health Professions Education 4*, 3–8.

4   Cruess, R. and Cruess, S. (1997) 'Professionalisms must be taught.' *British Medical Journal 315*, 1674–1677.

5   General Medical Council (2014) *Good Medical Practice*. Accessed on 15/2/2022 at www.gmc-uk.org/ethical-guidance/ethical-guidance-for-doctors/good-medical-practice.

6   Stick, H. (2000) 'Toward a normative definition of medical professionalism.' *Academic Medicine 200*, 75, 612–616.

7   Carina, S., Neumann, O., Baertschi, M. and Ritz, A. (2019) 'Public service motivation, prosocial motivation and altruism: Towards disentanglement and conceptual clarity.' *International Journal of Public Administration 42*, 14, 1200–1211.

8   Frey, B. S. and Jegen, R. (2001) 'Motivation Crowding Theory.' *Journal of Economic Surveys 15*, 5, 589–611.

9   Deci, E. L. (1971) 'Effects of externally mediated rewards on intrinsic motivation.' *Journal of Personality and Social Psychology 18*, 1, 105–115.

10   Standing, G. (2019) *Plunder of the Commons: A Manifesto for Sharing Public Wealth.* London: Pelican.

11   Titmuss, R. M. (1971) *The Gift Relationship.* London: Allen and Unwin.

12   Frey and Jegen (2001).

13   Fehr, E. and Falk, A. (2002) 'Psychological foundations of incentives.' *European Economic Review 46*, 687–724.

14   Frey, B. S. and Oberholzer-Gee, F. (1997) 'The cost of price incentives: An empirical analysis of motivation crowding-out.' *American Economic Review 87*, 4, 746–755.

15   Frey and Jegen (2001).

16   Mahon, A. (2013) 'Relationships in Healthcare.' In S. Llewellyn, S. Brookes and A. Mahon (eds), *Trust and Confidence in Government and Public Services.* London: Routledge.

17   Le Grand, J. (2003) *Motivation, Agency, and Public Policy: Of Knights and Knaves, Pawns and Queens.* Oxford: Oxford University Press.

18   Georgellis, Y., Iossa, E. and Tabvuma, V. (2009) *Crowding out Public Service Motivation.* Accessed on 15/2/2022 at https://bura.brunel.ac.uk/handle/2438/3922.

19   Bolino, M. C., Klotz, A. C., Turnley, W. H. and Harvey, J. (2013) 'Exploring the dark side of organizational citizenship behavior.' *Journal of Organizational Behavior 34*, 4, 542–559, p.542.

20   Van Dyne, L. and Ellis, J. B. (2004) 'Job creep: A reactance theory perspective on organizational citizenship behavior: Construct redefinition, measurement and validation.' *Academy of Management Journal 37*, 77–93.

21   Bolino *et al.* (2013), p.546.

22   Bolino *et al.* (2013).

23   *Ibid.*

24   Berdud, M., Cabasés, J. M. and Nieto, J. (2016) 'Incentives and intrinsic motivation in healthcare.' *Gaceta Sanitaria 30*, 6, 408–414.

Marion and Gordon

Community geriatricians have to learn their geography quite well: the challenge of finding patients' homes in small, rural villages inevitably leads to some exploring. Often, it's simpler to stop and ask for directions, but in the smaller villages, it's better to ask for the person than the house. The person giving directions will often direct you using useful local landmarks (postboxes, village halls and pubs are the best) and, not infrequently, they will also give you an update of the patient's medical condition.

No such localism was on show when I visited Marion. I knew the street her apartment was on, but I could not find the building. Eventually, I found it, nestled in the corner of a piece of land previously owned by the council and now sold for private development. Where once a lawn had been, to one side of the dilapidated but formerly grand register office, there now stood a modern construction of beige panels and windows, two stories high, squat and unremarkable. It was a new 'retirement village', which appeared to be a misappropriation of the term, to describe expensive but small, self-contained flats, available to retirees. Entry was via an intercom. There was no one present to let you in. One entered the building through large, pristine and entirely empty communal lounges. I suspected that residents were fearful of muddying the thick, cream carpets.

Marion and Gordon's flat was new, clean and small. Modern housing is often striking in its lack of storage space. They had also made the cardinal homebuyer's mistake of not buying furniture for the flat they were in, instead transporting it from the previous, much larger home.

They had moved to West Dorset from Birmingham. They had no connection with Dorset at all but had been lured by an advert in a paper. The cost of their new flat was half the value of their old house, and they liked the idea of freeing up capital to help out their children.

Marion had managed the move well. Her heart failure meant that she became breathless after 50 yards (that was why I was seeing her), so she spent most of her time indoors, indulging her passion for embroidery. She sewed, read books and chatted endlessly to their children and grandchildren on her iPad.

Gordon, however, was finding it difficult. When I asked him what he thought of Bridport, he told me that it didn't have any decent shops (it doesn't – but it does have a very good twice-weekly market). I told him that West Dorset was really about its connection with the sea and the countryside and asked him if he had explored anywhere nearby. He told me that he had been to Lyme Regis (9 miles away), Exeter (40 miles away) and Bristol (65 miles away).

My description of more local attractions (the beaches, best cafes and beauty spots) was politely acknowledged but clearly ignored.

Miles away from family and friends, Gordon was lost. A good retirement is never only about the nature of one's accommodation, and too often, we underplay the importance of the routines of daily life in finding our everyday meaning. I have met scores of people who sell their family homes on retirement and move to rural West Dorset. They may know the place from holidays but lack the roots that kept them anchored in the communities they have moved from. In early retirement, when they are fit and well, they often compensate for their aimlessness by travelling lots and having grandchildren to visit. As frailty mounts, however, they find themselves unable to drive and are marooned in the countryside, relying on neighbours and friends, but dislocated from the people they need the most – their families.

CHAPTER 11

Age Segregation

The bias of a professional life spent caring for older patients creates the impression that the demands of meeting the needs of an ageing population seem to fall at the feet of our medical services. The shape of our NHS is part of the answer, but it is not the most important.

Society is shaped by the healthcare system that serves it, but the reverse is also true. While the NHS has had a particular effect on our collective psyche, the values of society in general are enshrined in the people who work in the NHS. The insidious effect of our political landscape on our cultural and social values is difficult to quantify. For the moment, let us acknowledge only that it is there but leave it aside for a more artful focus on the current context of ageing in the UK, outside of politics.

Atul Gawande[1] comments that in India, his older relatives are looked after by their families. He is tempted to draw comparisons with the care of seniors he has witnessed in the United States, but a cursory glance at the population profiles for India compared with the UK (see Figures 1 and 2) indicates instantly where the comparison falls down.

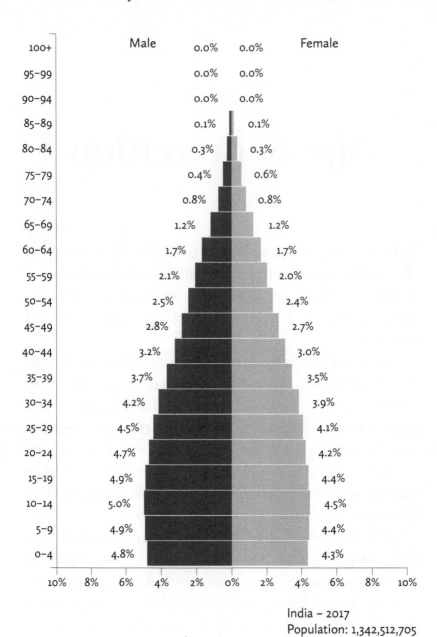

India – 2017
Population: 1,342,512,705

Figure 1

Source: PopulationPyramid.net[2]

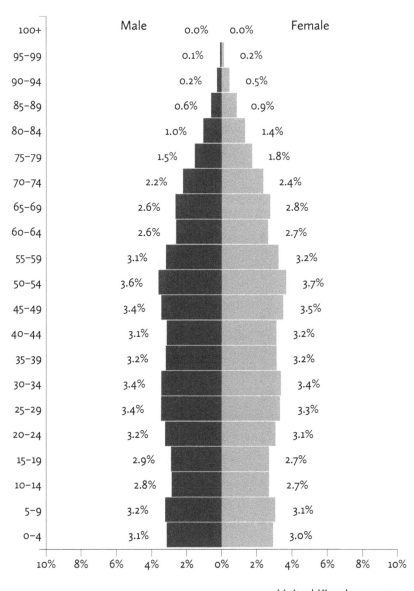

Figure 2

Source: PopulationPyramid.net[3]

Note its steadiness as age rises – we do not fall away with time as in India. As each band ripples upwards, undiminished, it takes with it the question of how the enduring presence of elders changes the normal functioning of our society. India lags behind us on this measure, and it is only beginning to discover the extent of societal modification required to accommodate a prevalent, ageing population. When I visited India in the mid-noughties, the average life expectancy was 67 years. It now stands at 68.5 years.[4] It was a challenge to explain to them the type of medicine I practised for a living – they did not understand the need for people like me.

In 1946, the National Insurance Act introduced a contributory state pension for everyone, which could be drawn at the age of 65.[5] The life expectancy at birth in 1950 was about 63 years for men.[6] Put briefly, one worked, and then one died. To modern sensibilities, it is an appalling notion. It is clear, however, that the concept of the third age is a new one for us, both as a species and as a society. Built into the origins of a universal state pension is the value judgement that if you survived long enough, you earned a supported dotage. I doubt that this is the prevalent sentiment that lingers today – retirement is the domain for active plans, forestalled by the realities and costs of mortgages, children and career development. It is dangerous to delay one's dreams, but our collective expectation is for time and resources to chase leisure and recreation. This is clearly a broad brush I am painting with, but consider the recent finding that younger generations today will have less wealth at every point in their lives than previous generations, and this will not be evened out by inheritance.[7]

The possible nature of retirement today should not over-influence one's expectation for retirement in the future. Baby Boomers now account for 36% of household wealth,[8] but the generations to come will be less well prepared for retired life: fewer millennials will ever be homeowners and, on average, will be 61 before they inherit their parents' wealth;[9] 40% of first-time buyers will still be paying off their mortgages when they reach the age of 65.[10] Even among today's pensioners, wealth is most unevenly distributed – 2.1 million pensioners live below the poverty line.[11] In a future with no final salary pensions, reduced home ownership, rising private rents[12] and flat incomes,[13] the prospects for the retired life of the future are looking bleak, even before one factors in the potential impacts on society in general from climate change and environmental degradation. At the least granular level of fortune telling, one can predict great changes over the next 50 years. Only a fool would predict their precise form, but even today, the early shoots of the difficulties ahead are visible in the lives and struggles of our elders.

Of the over-75s, 51% of live alone,[14] and 40% of older people report that the television is their main source of company.[15] Within the statistics, there are to be found the real stories: Elizabeth, a lady in her 80s who fell at home, was on the floor for four days before anyone found her. Unable to stand up, and wedged between her bed and her radiator, she developed burns from the radiator, a large pressure sore from the floor and, rather paradoxically given where she fell, a profound hypothermia: when I put my hand on her to feel her pulse, she was ice-cold. She died that day, which is sad enough, but sadder still is meeting someone whose isolation allowed her to lie on the floor for four days unnoticed by anyone.

Stories like Elizabeth's are unnervingly common. However, they are partially offset by heart-warming examples of the fulfilment of filial duty. Betty was a lady in her 80s with advanced dementia, looked after at home by her son. She was a frail lady, a tiny slip of a thing, who struggled to remain orientated in time or place – meaningful conversation was limited by her fragile concentration and her loosening grasp on reality. Events simply did not make sense to her for long enough to give her any context or meaning. Her son, however, acted as a conduit to reality, able to divine meaning and understanding from the intuition born out of close scrutiny of every sound, movement and clue. To Betty's son, caring was his full-time job – one to which he was committed – and his attentions showed. Betty was clean and well nourished and lived in a warm home surrounded by great affection. Betty experienced daily what it meant to be loved, and no amount of medicine can replace that. Without her son, Betty would have been in a nursing home and considerably more poorly.

Clearly, Betty benefited, and perhaps her care is the ideal we should all aim for. The cost of her care, however, was the hopes and ambitions of her son. A capable man in his mid-40s, his whole life was directed towards the needs of his ailing mother. Wider society benefited from the offset costs of otherwise caring for her, taken on at considerable discount by the son. Yet wider society lacked the contribution Betty's son could have made. He was clearly a capable carer, but what else could he have achieved without the responsibility for his mother?

Informal care is only fleetingly recognised by the health and social care system. The Office for National Statistics estimates that informal carers provide £57 billion of care.[16] The implication is that if they decided to down tools, we would be left to foot the bill. The reality of a mass informal-carer walkout would be the misery and neglect of a host of vulnerable people across the country. However, it is distasteful to boil it all down to money. It is always nice to get a bargain, but that rather misses the point: some of the uncounted cost of informal care is the removal of active community participants from general circulation and the recognition that the needs of the old and the frail require us to retire from the routines of society and deal with the challenges in private.

Think about the prospects for Betty's son: for the last ten years he had been fully invested in caring for his own mother. During that time, he had not pursued a career, he had not had his own family. What would he do when his mother died? What would his purpose be? Who would look after him when he was old and frail? It was not Betty's future I worried about. Betty's son deserved praise for his dedication and expertise in managing someone with complex dementia. He taught me that excellence is possible, but this also shines a spotlight on the cost of excellence within the framework of older people's care that we have established over the last generation.

The common theme across the wealth spectrum of ageing is that of segregation. Older people live apart and often alone. Almost 4 million people over the age of 65 live by themselves[17] and another half a million live in care homes.[18] Age UK estimated in 2016 that 1.2 million older people were unable to receive the care and support they needed.[19] Much of the care that older people need comes from spouses. There are over 2 million older carers in the UK, 400,000 of whom are over 80 years old.[20]

The reality of being old and frail in the UK is some distance from the image of Baby Boomers, enjoying endless leisure time on generous pensions, but for all the reasons given above, the future is much more stark.

Part of this reality has already been recognised: pension ages are rising, and costs of pensions are rising, becoming unaffordable for many, as doctors are currently discovering.[21] I doubt there is much sympathy from people outside of the public sector: the defined contribution pensions available to most people offer tax benefits but little else: you get back what you put in and hope for a good return on your investments over time. Auto-enrolment has improved the take-up of pensions savings,[22] but the Financial Conduct Authority estimates that 31% of people have no private pension provision and will therefore be relying entirely on the state pension for their subsistence in retirement.[23]

The emerging truth for many, therefore, is that retirement will be a graded process. Financial imperatives will mean that ongoing financial commitments (e.g. housing costs) and insufficient retirement funds will require many to continue working after retirement age. What is disappearing, therefore, is the expectation among professional staff that they will work a fixed-term career of about 30 years, at the end of which they will retire and not work. Already, times are changing – the Office for National Statistics estimates that there are

1.2 million people over the age of 65 in employment, up from half that number in 2006. [24]

The gradual transition of retirement from fortunate longevity to expectation has not been matched by sufficient modification of the nature of retirement over time. The complexity of managing an increasingly ageing and frail population is multifaceted, but one key moment is the transition into old age. Frailty emerges gradually, and by the time it takes grip, the lives of those affected have transitioned away from families and often from the communities they spent most of their lives working in.

Retirement as a cliff edge is the problem: the move from active participant in the workforce to pensioner is often too abrupt and at best unhelpful. Economic realities are making such retirements impractical, but there are other reasons to move away from them as well. The 'traditional' route to a pension is rooted in the idea of a linear career in which one rises to the apex of one's ability, where one remains until retirement. There is, therefore, the professional expectation that one retires at the height of one's authority and responsibility, and the promotion of younger employees requires the space above them to be vacated.

However, the notion of such a linear career has been weakened in recent times. Tania Luna and Jordan Cohen[25] argue that the idea of a career as being a straight journey to a final destination is a myth, outlining that 70% of employees feel there are insufficient opportunities for career progression, while 75% of organisations expect there to be a shortage of required skills and knowledge. The implication is that our traditional structures and hierarchies hinder us from developing staff at the rate and volume required. A modern focus on competencies and skills rather than responsibility is needed.

A graded retirement has a number of benefits – it retains skills and expertise within the workforce, and it encourages continued active participation in the economy and community. Universal pension ages seem inappropriate: an affluent male professional, who might be able to afford to retire early, can expect to live 11 years longer than a low-income manual labourer.[26] Modern demographics suggest at least an economic need for longer contribution to the labour market, but modern pension arrangements do not encourage it. It is likely that the individual wealth of the majority of retirees will diminish over time, and the demographic changes of the population suggest an increasing reliance on either a smaller number of younger people or a large number of older people, depending on your perspective.

Economic realities therefore suggest that people will have to work later into their lives, simply to afford the essential costs of life. However, for the purposes of meeting the needs of our most frail people, there is the potential for changing workforce structures to deliver positive benefits later in life.

In his 1961 book, *Asylums*, Ernest Goffman remarked that, 'a basic social arrangement in modern society is that the individual tends to sleep, play and work in different places'.[27] His observation is pertinent to the mechanisms by which we have sought to contain the challenge of ageing populations. Even independent living developments for retirees, but most notably care homes, hive off older people to live in isolation from the workings of wider society. Goffman highlights the tendency of 'total institutions'[28] to be symbolised by the 'barrier to social intercourse with the outside world'.[29] Warden-controlled flats may not be 'total institutions' the way care homes are, but they might be considered way points.

At this point in the discourse, we move more into the realms of supposition. We glanced at the upcoming economic horizons for future pensioners and acknowledged the extent of social isolation among the older people, as well as the relative scarcity of the home help they require. Add on to these data points the evidence that loneliness is associated with higher mortality,[30] and that the Institute of Economic Affairs suggests that retirement itself can be associated with deteriorations in physical and mental health.[31] Maintaining independent function is the goal of many interventions for older patients, and it is a magic-free zone: rehabilitation and adaptation are the cornerstones of recovery and preservation of independence in geriatric practice. Frailty is often the component that contributes most to poor recovery from illness.

Frailty is considered in medical circles to be a long-term condition in its own right; it cannot be cured but there is some evidence that it can be modified.[32] The science is still nascent, but Ostir *et al.* contend that a positive affect is associated with slower progression of frailty.[33] At present, the management of frailty focuses on its early identification, expert management of associated long-term conditions and, in more advanced cases, planning in advance the goals for medical intervention.

Rates of social isolation and depression among older people are high. These are both modifiable, through social innovation rather than medical intervention. We remain mortal beings, with time-limited lives, but the details of those lives can be influenced. One aspect of managing an ageing population successfully necessarily centres on maximising the number of years spent in good health and reducing the number of years in poor health prior to death.

Loneliness is the symptom, but segregation is the disease. By the time frailty takes hold, and dependence takes grip, older couples, widows and widowers find themselves removed from family, removed from the activity of normal life. The lucky ones have neighbours, friends and families to help them out, but what jars is the sense that senescence takes place away from the mainstream.

Intergenerational interactions are a classic win-win: older people demonstrate improvements in physical, emotional and cognitive affect,[34] while younger participants improve social behaviour as well as perceptions and attitudes to ageing.[35] Yet outside of grandparent relationships, little is done to integrate the lives of the old and the young. One does not need peer-reviewed articles to understand the restorative effect of children on older people, one only needs to visit a care home or hospital ward with a small child to see it. There are a range of efforts to enforce familiarity, well represented by endeavours such as Channel 4's *Old People's Home for 4 Year Olds*. However, these bear the hallmarks of tokenism, inspired by good intentions but made necessary by the habits of the present, in which older people live partitioned off from the rest of us.

Our failure to create a niche within our daily lives for our elders is to the detriment of all of us. We used to rely on older people as sources of knowledge, wisdom and tradition, but now the internet has become our centralised knowledge repository, we deny ourselves the prism of experience to make sense of the past. There is nothing like the perspective of today's elders to give one's own problems context: the privations of growing up in the 1920s and 1930s, as well as the struggle of the Second World War – in fact, almost any aspect of the past – can serve as a useful counterpoint to the present. Older people serve as a gentle reminder that life is finite, and their perspective on what is important to us, at the end of a long life, may well differ from what you worry about today.

I often remember Clifford, a 97-year-old man, who had been married to his 92-year-old wife for 72 years. 'Still getting to know her, son!' is what he would say. This is not a reflection of his capacity for learning but rather an example of his boundless energy and kindness. Contrast him with Alfred, a man in his 80s, who lived a life of desperate loneliness and sadness. His misfortune (at least in the 1950s) was to realise he was gay. He spent his adult life in a mixture of secrecy and guilt. The only way he could hide his true nature from his family was to separate himself from them – he had not seen his siblings in decades. And all the while he felt ashamed of himself. He never found love and never enjoyed intimate companionship. He had few friends and never forgave himself for being homosexual. He died alone at home, unloved and unmissed. We cannot rewind our lives, but we can pay attention to the lessons of others, if only we give ourselves the chance to see.

Perhaps it lacks drama to take this moral and relate it back to the way we retire, but this is only the starting point. Ignorance of ageing is one problem and ignorance of the value of older people is another. The integration of ageing into mainstream society activity starts with valuing experience forged over time. Stamina wanes, but experience grants perspective, and intergenerational collaboration breeds familiarity and openness. It is not benevolence to invite older people to remain active participants in the workplace or in communities – it is good practice. For it is the presence of meaning and purpose that underpins mental and even physical health. Well-functioning societies are both inclusive and appreciative. Older people may not be able to work in the same way as they used to – indeed, I doubt they want to. The workplace, however, makes little provision for retaining the experience and input of people who have plenty still to offer, if we had the wherewithal to adapt to their needs. We do not miss older people in the workplace, simply because we have not really experienced it. One cannot miss what one has never had.

The economic imperatives for later retirement are clear, but isn't it nicer to know that working later in our lives would do us all some good? It is up to us to create the professional and social context in which the continued contributions of older workers are encouraged, but at the outset, it starts with our mindset.

People will still become unwell and frail, but they will do so from a position of greater social inclusion. We will be more familiar with the sights and sounds of ageing, more appreciative of the challenges and more able to support the difficulties through the simple expedient of being more familiar. It is not the total solution, only a first step in recognising the challenge of meeting the needs of frail strangers disengaged from the usual functioning of society.

Endnotes

1   Gawande, A. (2014) *Being Mortal: Illness, Medicine and What Matters in the End.* London: Wellcome Collection.

2   PopulationPyramid.net (2019) *Population Pyramids of the World from 1950 to 2100.* Accessed on 17/2/2022 at www.populationpyramid.net.

3   PopulationPyramid.net (2019) *Population Pyramids of the World from 1950 to 2100.* Accessed on 17/2/2022 at www.populationpyramid.net.

4   The World Bank (2017) *Life Expectancy at Birth, Total (Years).* Accessed on 17/2/2022 at https://data.worldbank.org/indicator/sp.dyn.le00.in.

5   Tetlow, G., Crawford, R. and Bozio, A. (2010) *The History of State Pensions in the UK: 1948 to 2010. IFS Briefing Note BN105.* Institute for Fiscal Studies. Accessed on 17/2/2022 at www.ifs.org.uk/bns/bn105.pdf.

6   Office for National Statistics (2015) *How Has Life Expectancy Changed Over Time?* Accessed on 17/2/2022 at www.ons.gov.uk/peoplepopulationandcommunity/birthsdeathsandmarriages/lifeexpectancies/articles/howhaslifeexpectancychangedovertime/2015-09-09.

7   Crossley, T. and O'Dea, C. (2016) *The Distribution of Household of Wealth in the UK.* Institute for Fiscal Studies. Accessed on 17/2/2022 at www.ifs.org.uk/publications/8239.

8   Asgaria, N. (2019) 'One in five UK baby boomers are millionaires.' *Financial Times.* Accessed on 17/2/2022 at www.ft.com/content/c69b49de-1368-11e9-a581-4ff78404524e.

9   Resolution Foundation (2018) *A New Generational Contract: The Final Report of the Intergenerational Commission.* The Resolution Foundation. Accessed on 17/2/2022 at www.resolutionfoundation.org/advanced/a-new-generational-contract.

10 Collinson, P. (2019) 'Four in 10 UK first-time buyers will retire with mortgages, FCA warns.' *The Guardian.* Accessed on 17/2/2022 at www.theguardian.com/money/2019/jan/10/four-in-10-uk-first-time-buyers-will-retire-with-mortgages-fca-warns.

11 Age UK (2021) *Poverty in Later Life.* Accessed on 18/2/2022 at www.ageuk.org.uk/globalassets/age-uk/documents/policy-positions/money-matters/poverty_in_later_life_briefing_june_2021.pdf.

12 Joyce, R., Mitchell, M. and Norris-Keillor, A. (2017) *The Cost of Housing for Low Income Renters.* Institute for Fiscal Studies. Accessed on 17/2/2022 at www.ifs.org.uk/uploads/publications/comms/R132.pdf.

13 O'Conner, S. (2018) 'Millennials poorer than previous generations, data show.' *Financial Times.* Accessed on 17/2/2022 at www.ft.com/content/81343d9e-187b-11e8-9e9c-25c814761640.

14 Campaign to End Loneliness (n.d.) *Loneliness Research.* Accessed on 17/2/2022 at www.campaigntoendloneliness.org/loneliness-research.

15 Bolton, M. (2012) *Loneliness – The State We're In.* Age UK. Accessed on 17/2/2022 at www.campaigntoendloneliness.org/wp-content/uploads/Loneliness-The-State-Were-In.pdf.

16 Office for National Statistics (2017) *Unpaid Carers Provide Social Care Worth £57 Billion*. Office for National Statistics. Accessed on 17/2/2022 at www.ons.gov.uk/peoplepopulationandcommunity/healthandsocialcare/healthandlifeexpectancies/articles/unpaidcarersprovidesocialcareworth57billion/2017-07-10.

17 Statista (2017) *Number of People Living Alone in the United Kingdom (UK) 2017 by Age and Gender (in 1,000)*. Accessed on 17/2/2022 at www.statista.com/statistics/281616/people-living-alone-in-the-united-kingdom-uk-by-age-and-gender.

18 Age UK (2018) *Later Life in the United Kingdom*. Accessed on 17/2/2022 at www.ageuk.org.uk/globalassets/age-uk/documents/reports-and-publications/later_life_uk_factsheet.pdf.

19 Age UK (2018).

20 Age UK (2019) *Briefing: Health and Care of Older People in England 2019*. Accessed on 7/3/2022 at www.ageuk.org.uk/globalassets/age-uk/documents/reports-and-publications/reports-and-briefings/health--wellbeing/age_uk_briefing_state_of_health_and_care_of_older_people_july2019.pdf.

21 Dumbo, J. (2018) 'Budget pensions move could deepen doctor hiring crisis, says BMA.' *Financial Times*. Accessed on 17/2/2022 at www.ft.com/content/882bd322-d6a9-11e8-a854-33d6f82e62f8.

22 Department for Work and Pensions (2017) *Automatic Enrolment Review 2017: Analytical Report*. Accessed on 17/2/2022 at https://assets.publishing.service.gov.uk/government/uploads/system/uploads/attachment_data/file/668657/automatic-enrolment-review-2017-analytical-report.pdf.

23 Financial Conduct Authority (2018) *The Financial Lives of Consumers across the UK: Key Findings from the FCA's Financial Lives Survey 2017*. Accessed on 17/2/2022 at www.fca.org.uk/publication/research/financial-lives-consumers-across-uk.pdf.

24 Office for National Statistics (2018) *UK Labour Market: September 2018*. Accessed on 17/2/2022 at www.ons.gov.uk/employmentandlabourmarket/peopleinwork/employmentandemployeetypes/bulletins/uklabourmarket/september2018#summary-of-latest-labour-market-statistics.

25 Luna, T. and Cohen J. (2018) 'How to mentor someone who doesn't know what their career goals should be.' *Harvard Business Review*. Accessed on 17/2/2022 at https://hbr.org/2018/07/how-to-mentor-someone-who-doesnt-know-what-their-career-goals-should-be.

26 Harper, S., Howse, K. and Baxter, S. (2011) *Living Longer and Prospering? Designing an Adequate, Sustainable and Equitable UK State Pension System*. Oxford: Oxford Institute of Ageing.

27 Goffman, E. (1961) *Asylums: Essays on the Social Situation of Mental Patients and Other Inmates*. New York: Anchor Books, p.17.

28 *Ibid.*, p.16.

29 *Ibid.*, p.15.

30 Tilvis, R. S., Laitala, V., Routasalo, P. E. and Pitkälä, K. H. (2011) 'Suffering from loneliness indicates significant mortality risk of older people.' *Journal of Aging Research*, 534781.

31 Sahlgren, G. H. (2013) *Work Longer, Live Healthier: The Relationship Between Economic Activity, Health and Government Policy*. Institute of Economic Affairs. Accessed on 17/2/2022 at https://iea.org.uk/wp-content/uploads/2016/07/Work%20Longer,%20Live_Healthier.pdf.

32 Partridge, J., Harari, D. and Dhesi, J. K. (2012) 'Frailty in the older surgical patient: A review.' *Age and Ageing 41*, 2, 142–147.

33 Ostir, G. V., Ottenbacher, K. J. and Markides, K. S. (2004) 'Onset of frailty in older adults and the protective role of positive affect.' *Psychology of Ageing 19*, 3, 402–408.

34 George, D. R. and Wagner, G. (2014) 'Social learning and innovation: Developing two shared-site intergenerational reading programs in Hershey, Pennsylvania.' *Journal of Intergenerational Relationships 12*, 1, 69–74.

35 Kessler, E. and Staudinger, U. M. (2007) 'Intergenerational potential: Effects of social interaction between older adults and adolescents.' *Psychology and Aging 22*, 4, 690–704.

Wilfred

Wilfred is in his mid-90s. He is plagued by osteoarthritis. Osteo-arthritis is the type of arthritis that is usually characterised as the one that's due to wear and tear. While that remains broadly apt, it is sometimes better appreciated as an active inflammatory condition, where overuse or strain can cause flare-ups of pain and limited movement.

I say this only out of interest rather than it being of direct relevance to Wilfred. His osteoarthritis is both extensive and severe: extensive in the number of joints affected and severe in the degree to which his joints are diseased.

To look at one of his hip X-rays, for example, is to induce a strong sense of vicarious pain. You can see the ball of his hip joint rubbing into the socket, where normally there would be a black line of cartilage buffering the connection. The strong physical reaction to his X-rays is only amplified by seeing, and hearing, him stand up. It is a chorus of grunts, groans, creaking and cracking, resulting, eventually, in him stooping over his walking frame. His left foot is turned alarmingly outwards, and his knees bow inwards so that they rub together at each passing. Over time, this has rubbed away the skin on the inner aspect of his knees, leaving him with painful sores.

Joint replacement, for example of the hips and the knees, is primarily a treatment for pain. Wilfred would benefit from joint replacement, if it weren't for the fact that it would be too great an undertaking to replace all his diseased joints. Furthermore, the risk of an operation needs to be considered: his risk of dying is about 5–10%, but his risk of significant complication is about 33%. Given that multiple operations would need to be done to give him significant relief, no surgeon is prepared to consider him. In addition, his frailty jeopardises his physical recovery, meaning that he may well end up less mobile.

Wilfred is resigned to not having an operation. I referred him to the orthopaedic surgeon to discuss. It is important that patients do not feel that options for them have not been considered at all.

Despite the excruciating pain he suffers, and the ever-decreasing boundaries of his world (he has not been out of his house in a year) he remains a bright, engaging person. He occupies his mind with challenging books, writes letters to his friends and has embraced technology to video-call his children and grandchildren abroad.

His wife died some years ago from dementia and he commented to me that he was pleased that dementia has not robbed him of 'who I really am'.

He is still prone to moments of despair and recently asked me, 'What have I got to look forward to?' I demurred, spouting some line about only being a doctor and not the arbiter of personal meaning. It was not my proudest moment. Yet, he does not feel sorry for himself – at least not openly. I suspect he has dark moments in private, particularly first thing in the morning, when he is trying to drag his stiff, aching body out of bed.

CHAPTER 12

Perspective

Previous chapters reflect on the need for a more gradual glide into old age. The last chapter in particular highlights cliff-edge retirements, which result in the precipitous segregation of older people from mainstream routines. Social isolation in advanced age, in other words, can be traced back to the impact of decisions made some years earlier.

At present, society lacks both a purpose for older people and an appreciation for them. Evidence already highlighted outlines the positive benefits all round of intergenerational interactions. Yet, there are structural problems with modern professional, family and retired life that remove the routine opportunities for intergenerational congregations as a matter of normal routine.

Part of the thesis is that the successful care of the very frail begins with better stewardship of the transition into senescence, with the preservation of meaning as an important goal – something that is built on better husbandry of the role of the middle-aged and older people in the routine occurrences of ordinary life. Chapter 11 developed the concept that at retirement age, people have a great deal to offer in the workplace, as well as the requirement to remain in employment: the golden generation of retirement has passed, and the economic uncertainties of the future make sudden total retirements less affordable and plausible for most.

At the heart of the matter is the extent to which we collectively have adapted individually to myriad changes in the shape and function of our family lives over the last 50 years. A great deal has changed: from increasing longevity, changes in birth rates and the age of first-time mothers to numbers of women in the workplace, levels of home ownership, university attendance and the distribution of capital.

This brief summary is offered only as a contextual starting point to this question: 'While a great deal has changed, how well have we adapted?' Consider for a moment how the workplace has opened up to women, but then consider also whether it has adapted to them. There is still a gender pay gap, and who would make their last stand defending the idea that opportunities for women are not affected by their gender? Caroline Criado Perez highlights the multiple ways the modern world still operates around the needs of men in her book *Invisible Women*.[1]

It is not equality to expect women to choose families or careers when such a choice does not affect men. It is also self-defeating: a successful modern, liberal society seeks to support all citizens to achieve the best they are capable of. Yuval Harari[2] characterises liberal democracies as those that seek to enhance peace and prosperity through the provision and protection of individual liberties. It is also, as he points out, an imperfect experiment.

The point is that adaptation to significant societal changes invites focus on the issues that really matter. It is easy to focus on easy issues, but what are the issues that matter most? Much of the modern rhetoric still lands on the factors encapsulated on the level of safety in Maslow's hierarchy of needs[3] – financial, personal, health and personal security. Yet the manner in which we attend to these needs gives lie to our perception of what is really important. Remaining on Maslow for a moment, the pinnacle of his characterisation of existence is 'self-actualisation' – that is the achievement of one's full potential, which once the practical matters of existence have been mastered, lands on the global goal of finding happiness. Importantly, self-actualisation is self-defined and therefore varies significantly between people.

Although Maslow is a useful touchstone, his work is not a philosophical straightjacket: progression through his hierarchy need not be linear, and indeed, evidence suggests it is not. Tay and Diener[4] report that although people found that Maslow's hierarchy correlates quite well with the factors required for self-reported positive emotions about life, the completion of one level of need was not a prerequisite for success on a 'higher' level. It is possible to be poor and fulfilled, just as it is possible to be rich and unhappy. It's an interesting question to ponder: is it better to be happy and poor or rich and miserable?

The relationship between happiness and wealth, however, is more nuanced. Lyubomirsky and King argue that happiness not only follows on from success but also precedes it:[5] happy people do better, suggesting that there is a two-way flow between happiness and success.

Indeed, older people have something to teach us about contentment: Laura Carstensen[6] finds that as people age, they become happier and that how we use our time depends on how much time we think we all have. Her resulting Socioeconomic Selectivity Theory posits that shorter time horizons become an important source of motivation: the less time we have, the more we prioritise emotional goals – a challenge to the usual assumption made by younger people: that old age is a time of sadness and loss.

Carstensen is not trying to say that the emotional lives of older people are routinely happy – indeed, they are frequently not. Instead she is telling us that older people have richer emotional responses to meaningful activities. Of course, the emergence of contentment in old age may not itself be a function of age but instead of historical timing: for example, our current elders may actually be more miserable than we are, but they come from a heritage of stoicism that encourages them to put a brave face on suffering, perhaps because they have a better sense of what real suffering is. Alternatively, it is possible that old people today, the Silent Generation, who followed on from the Generation of the Second World War, have always had richer emotional lives, forged as they were by the impacts of the Great Depression and the Second World War.

Whatever the explanation, the key issue is perspective: the closer we are to dying, the more we attend to our emotional needs. The further away we are from bad events, the more positively we remember them. With this tendency to positivity comes also a tendency to poignancy: older people tend not to be rigidly positive about all things but instead mix together wistfulness and sadness with gratitude and happiness, and they do so in the context of greater emotional stability. So, while time may give us nostalgia, it also teaches us more stable emotional regulation: the emotional lives of older people appear to be less labile, and Carstensen's argument is that the co-existence of both positive and negative experiences delivers emotional stability, while emotional stability delivers an improved sense of well-being.

Contemporary experience of older people often reveals a grounded sense of purpose from the past they lived through: I met a man a few years ago who earnestly believed that the happiest years of his life were the time spent as a teenager in the Hitler Youth in the run-up to the Second World War. Perhaps if Germany had won, that sentiment would not jar so much, but what he alludes to is the memory of purpose and camaraderie. It was a period of his life when he knew what he was doing and why he was doing it, and identified with those around him. Nothing later came close to achieving that for him.

I have found a similar memory of purpose and meaning in men and women who lived through the Blitz or fought in the war. One capable lady told me of the time she came back to London at the height of the bombings and was thrilled to live in a city so devastated, yet united, by its daily perils.

A ward round a few months ago was delayed by the drawn out but utterly compelling story a gentleman told me of his time in the Navy in the Far East. With a forensic memory of detail, but almost without any emotional embellishment, he told a story of a Japanese torpedo detonating near, but not on, his ship. In the aftermath, as they assessed the minimal damage, they eventually realised that the ship's doctor had not been seen. The gentleman was sent to the medical bay and described with eerie dispassion finding the man entirely unscathed except for the fact that he was in two pieces. They surmised that he had been chopped in half by the blast wave of the torpedo.

I recount his story not for the facts of the case but for the manner of its telling. A great many patients of mine bore the scars of their experiences and losses from the Second World War, but at the same time bore the memories of defeating an existential threat as a nation with pride.

What these people project is the concurrent presence of regret and pride. It harks back to the point that Carstensen makes about the wistfulness that accompanies old age but also the emotional stability that occurs in the presence of positive and negative experiences. The grounding effect of meaning and purpose rings out also. They lived through seminal times and their efforts through a period of great change were rewarded eventually by living through times of great progress and prosperity.

The need for meaning seems to exist in all of us and is perhaps embodied by Maslow's self-actualisation. Perhaps the magnitude of our collective achievements in the Second World War resonated across the decades, and the patients who related to me their stories were really telling me that it was those experiences that allowed, and justified, everything that followed.

Their misfortune was to live through the most devastating war in human history. Their luck was that it secured forever for them the meaning of their lives. One should not need events of this magnitude in order to have meaning, but one definitely needs meaning. One also needs perspective: how one interprets events is influenced by the frame of reference, and older people have a wider field of view.

Each era has its important moments, but the 21st Century seemed benign and low-key compared to the 20th Century, until the COVID pandemic. Contemporary events reveal some of the unifying effect of shared purpose and threat. To imagine the perfect liberal ideal is to risk imagining the society of Huxley's *Brave New World*, in which, lest we forget, most people are perfectly contented. Orson Welles was in a similar mode in *The Third Man*, when he remarked that the Borgias stewarded 30 years of blood and terror, which spawned 'Michelangelo, Leonardo and the Renaissance' while Switzerland enjoyed five centuries of 'democracy and brotherly love', which gave us the cuckoo clock.

Here and now, at the beginning of the 21st Century, we are in the middle of the most peaceful era of human history. Our blitheness has been shaken by the pandemic and will be further shaken by global heating, but we have yet to figure out how we are going to adjust. Before us lies the choice of how we find meaning. Is it through difference or conflict, or are we able, as a species, to adapt? Grounds for optimism are limited. We are witnessing a rising tide of resurgent populism manifesting in boldly anti-factual positions: think of Trump and Brexit. Superimpose the prevailing winds of climate change and environmental degradation, and now, coronavirus, and one begins to see the spectre of mass starvation and migration beginning to coalesce. Would you predict that we can address these issues collectively and intelligently?

In a global world, the web of co-dependencies for many of the normal functions of everyday society are so complex and interwoven that we cannot begin to dissect them all and deal with them on a national basis. And still we lack the maturity and mechanisms for dealing with global issues on a supranational basis. This absence is being felt right now in our uncoordinated global response to COVID-19.

The modern religion of capitalism is revealing its fundamental flaws: wealth flows preferentially to the wealthy[7] and no society can grow indefinitely without bursting through the limits of what the Earth can sustain. Capitalism does not equip us with the tools required to take a global view on addressing the issues that threaten our planet and its existence. Those hoping for technological solutions to our problems are outsourcing their agency rather than owning their own impact on the world.

Either by necessity (through catastrophic climate change, environmental degradation and subsequent social upheaval) or choice, we are faced with a future of simpler lives and simpler choices. Quality of life will be described less by what the GDP is doing, or how many units Apple shifts, and more in terms of the quality of our social and personal lives. Yuval Harari predicts unprecedented changes in the next 50 years, not just through the effects of our lives on the Earth, but also through the effects on our lives of technological change, such as Artificial Intelligence (AI). AI is set to become better than we are at most things, perhaps even creativity. The cycle of technological change will mean that in each person's life, the nature of what they do with their life – what they spend their time doing – will change every 10–20 years. Jobs done by people will increasingly be automated and improved upon by AI, which leaves the fundamental question, 'What are we for?'

Thus, the question that currently spoils the lives of our elders is likely to spoil the lives of all of us. In a world where you cannot usefully perform any function, how will you find meaning? Allied to the probability that in this same world, we will have to live lives with smaller carbon footprints, the size of the task is doubled.

The impact of the human race on the Earth has been fuelled by our ability to cooperate across populations and distances, usually under the banner of shared ideology. This has, at various times, been mythology, kin and kingship, but the overbearing influence over the last 2000 years has been religion. Capitalism and money have been the prevalent forces since the Industrial Revolution, but it will not see us through the next 100 years successfully without adaptation: contemporary capitalism is founded on the need for relentless growth, and our environmental impact is already showing us that there be dragons further along this path.

The needs of the future are made more daunting by the complexity of the issues that we have to grapple with. The reality of our lives is that by ourselves, we are capable of very little. It is only as members of a coordinated whole that we exert a positive effect. NASA estimates that it took 400,000 people to land a man on the moon.[8] Our motivational ideology has to adapt to reflect the global need for collaboration, or we will fail at the task.

Thus, for all our fantasies, we each exist as a tiny pocket of irrelevance when compared against the whole of existence. Within such a dispiriting conclusion, however, lies the key. I recall a 'No Fear' slogan from my teenage years, which stated, 'He who dies with the most toys, still dies.' After all, for all the advances of modern life, we are still mortal flesh, and the simplest and most profound marker of a life well lived is a death met with contentment and readiness.

The concept of a good death is real, but it is also subjective. We die in just as many ways as we live. Contentment grows out of a sense of meaning and purpose fulfilled. The bias of modern life is the pretence that none of us is mortal and that each of us is important. The bare truth is that while each of us is unique, none of is special – the only certainty that we are each born with is that we will die.

But I can relate to you countless stories of people who face death with calmness and readiness, and the sense that they have done everything they meant to. Meaning for them was found at home, with their spouse of decades, in their children in whose achievements they found great pride, in their successes and in their failures. Those who died with the most money, or houses, or cars, still died.

It is older people who can potentially remind us of the circumspection about existence that modern life takes away from us. A life spent in the company of the aged is a life spent aware of the frailties and impermanence of existence, with the benefits of experience and perspective. The current structure of modern society denies older people of the one function they can fulfil – it is not wisdom they necessarily offer us but the wide angle of life viewed from the perspective of many decades.

In our lives today we consciously refuse to be grounded by the needs of our frail relatives: the horizons for human potential seem endless, and who wants to be anchored down at home? However, the era of relentless progress is ending: technological change will continue apace, but change is coming in the form of economic limitations and the need for sustainability. The change may be enforced, but there is a positive angle to the difference: perhaps holding us back is the one favour older people can do for us. In a world addicted to unsustainable growth and consumerism, older people serve as a constant reminder that we, as individuals, only make sense as part of our narrative histories. Each of us is a unique collection of our experiences and environment, and is forged out of the unbroken history of our heritage. The task of caring for our elders is the first part of reminding ourselves that we have no mission statement. Existence is what we make it, and our fundamental duty lies with those around us.

The cost or challenge of care provision for older people is an issue that ought to be tackled. Failure to do so will result in significant suffering. Yet, it is futile to hope for a future in which older people can be looked after by their families: changes in demography, economics and family structures make it impossible for the solution to be a restoration of the past. Instead, we need to look to multifaceted solutions that address structural and social issues that make the challenge harder to manage. In the final chapters, we will look at the social and economic issues that feed into some of the problems I have outlined about ageing. One should appreciate that many of the problems and challenges relating to old age are not purely problems of old age but, instead, issues that are exaggerated by how modern society is structured and operates. The symptoms are in the nature of old age, but the causes lie in the generic habits and policies of modern society.

Endnotes

1   Criado Perez, C. (2020) *Invisible Women: Exposing Data Bias in a World Designed for Men*. London: Vintage.

2   Harari, Y. (2018) *21 Lessons for the 21st Century*. London: Vintage.

3   Maslow, A. H. (1943) 'A theory of human motivation.' *Psychological Review 50*, 4, 370–396.

4   Tay, L. and Diener, E. (2011) 'Needs and subjective well-being around the world.' *Journal of Personality and Social Psychology 101*, 2, 354–365.

5   Lyubomirsky, S. and King, L. (2005) 'The benefits of frequent positive affect: Does happiness lead to success?' *Psychological Bulletin 131*, 6, 803–855.

6   Carstensen, L. L., Turan, B., Scheibe, S., Ram, N. *et al.* (2011) 'Emotional experience improves with age: Evidence based on over 10 years of experience sampling.' *Psychology and Aging 26*, 1, 21–33.

7   Piketty, T. (2014) *Capital in the Twenty-First Century*. Cambridge: Harvard University Press.

8   Riley, C. (2009) 'The 400,000 strong backup team.' *The Guardian*. Accessed on 18/2/2022 at www.theguardian.com/science/2009/jul/02/apollo-11-back-up-team.

Bruce

When I met Bruce, he was already of advanced age, with severe bronchiectasis and heart failure. Bruce broadcast his years on his weathered face and in his wheezing, which signalled any form of physical effort. Bronchiectasis is a chronic lung condition in which the fine air sacs deep in the lungs become mucus factories, transforming them from islands of gas exchange into incubators for infections. The life of the bronchiectactic is one of deteriorating breathing, punctuated by episodes of even worse breathlessness during the bouts of frequent infection. The recovery from each infection is generally incomplete, and the relapsing-remitting pattern of acute infections is compounded by the underlying deterioration of the lungs over time.

As Bruce's lungs failed, so too did his heart. He experienced the progressive accumulation of water in his lungs and his legs from his fading cardiovascular system. Bruce oscillated uncomfortably between the breathlessness of a man coughing relentlessly and the breathlessness of a man slowly drowning in his own lungs. Understandably, he started sleeping in his armchair, where he could remain comfortably upright, in the sitting room of his house. I call it his house, except, according to the law, it no longer was.

Twelve years previously, in a moment of beneficence he would come to regret, he had gifted the house to his son. They lived together in an uneasy entente. For Bruce, it was the one meaningful gesture he could make to his son – he never expected to live this long, and it seemed both macabre and drawn out to make his son wait for him to die in order to inherit the house. There was no other way that Ryan, his son, would have been able to afford a family home of his own. For Ryan, it seemed like a fair deal: early inheritance on the understanding that his father could live out his days with him.

But the reality of caring for someone with chronic medical problems is a great deal harder than the idea of doing it. To begin with, it was the little things that upset Ryan the most – the incessant hacking cough, the monopoly on the television. Then it was the stubbornness: Ryan offered to convert the garage downstairs into a bedroom for his father, but Bruce refused. To him, accepting living in a downstairs bedroom was an admission of defeat. In the same vein, Bruce refused to use a walking stick or a Zimmer frame, and suffered a number of falls. The injuries were never serious, but Bruce spent more and more time downstairs, and Ryan found himself caring for an ever more frail old man.

There is a very great difference between being someone's carer and their son – the latter asks for love, perhaps even deference, while the former calls for a matter-of-fact intimacy with the most basic of human functions. Ryan was poorly suited to the role of carer, but it was not this that drove him from his father.

Instead, it was the unacknowledged inversion of the power dynamics that really drove them apart. For, although Bruce was a frail, old man, and Ryan was now running the farm they lived on, Bruce still treated Ryan the way he had always done: he criticised Ryan's plans for the next season on the farm, and at the end of every day, when Ryan came in from working, Bruce gave him a list of tasks he wanted Ryan to do for him.

Ryan was able to hold his tongue and ensure that his father was well cared for, but the tipping point was when Bruce started sleeping in the living room. This meant that there was nowhere for Ryan to sit down and unwind at the end of his long day of labour. It wasn't just that his dad was always there, it was also that his dad was always there and coughing away, wiping his phlegm into a dirty rag he kept stuffed down the side of his easy chair.

It is impossible to tell if Ryan's action was premeditated or simply opportunistic. One morning, while out in the yard, he heard his father calling out for help. In the living room, Ryan found him on the floor, struggling for breath and soiled. The ambulance arrived within 30 minutes, and within an hour, Bruce was on his way to hospital. It was the last time he would see the farm.

A week later, Ryan took a call from the hospital, informing him that his dad was ready to go home. Ryan told the ward sister who had called him that his father was no longer welcome to live in his house, and they would have to sort something else out for him.

'It's my house, and I should get to decide who lives here,' he explained.

Bruce spent another six weeks in hospital, while social services assessed his finances and eventually found him a nursing home, where he died three months later.

CHAPTER 13

The Wider Perspective

Old age does not have a starting point. We drift into it. Problems that find their expression in our later lives have often been seeded years or even decades before. Loneliness flows, for example, from the dramatic changes to family structures in the last 50 years; poverty is influenced by opportunities and financial decisions throughout one's working life. Physical health in our later years is heavily influenced by the environment we grew up in. Viewed in this way, to sandbox the experience of being old from everything that comes before is to deny our power to influence our lives through positive societal changes.

For example, I find inspiration in people who defy convention and time – the 90-year-old man who rides a motorbike or the woman in her 80s who completed a sociology degree to satisfy her curiosity. These are examples that defy convention but also confirm the bias that we expect old age to be a time for stagnation and regression. Too often we consider the lives of older people in isolation from the younger people they never stopped being.

Our cultural views on what it means to grow old forestall our ability to create a positive context for ageing. Hagestad and Uhlenberg,[1] for example, suggest that some of the expression of ageism derives from social structures that assign people of different ages to different social institutions. Kohli[2] argues that over the last 200 years, we have shifted from a categorical classification of people (what they do) to a temporal one (how old they are).

In cohorting each other by age, we create 'otherness' – older people become a tribe apart. In Chapter 11, I commented on the benefits of intergenerational interactions for both old and young, yet it is apparent that we have taken steps to engineer out of our lives the opportunities for such interactions to happen. In fact, age segregation has been so complete and so profound that we consider it normal. It was not always thus: Jared Diamond[3] describes how traditional communities spread the responsibility for child-rearing among the adults of a tribe (who are functionally an extended family) and how children grow up spending a lot of time observing what they do. Adults are familiar with children and children are familiar with adults, and the regular interplay between people of all ages renders age less important a fact. This is highlighted not as a template to define what is 'right' but to highlight that alternative societal structures are a reality.

Of course, ageing does bring changes, both physical and cognitive, but such changes are not grounds for segregation. It is the segregation of people by age, throughout society, that ultimately feeds into the loneliness and social isolation of our oldest and frailest neighbours. Pasupathi and Lochenhoff[4] usefully distinguish between ageist behaviour deriving from stereotypes and prejudices, and age-differentiated behaviour deriving from age-appropriate accommodation of age. There is a 'cycle of reproduction'[5] between age segregation and ageism that both reinforces its practice and further alienates different age cohorts.

The creation of a third age of retirement – of a demographic apart – for recreation and leisure has emerged only in the last few generations. While the prospect of a retirement may seem normal to us now, we should add context to our expectations by appreciating that it is a historical outlier. The expectation, or right, to a leisurely retirement is an illusion, perhaps born of hubris. More broadly, our current form of social striation is neither permanent nor compulsory. My great-grandparents never expected a fun retirement, and nor, I suspect, did yours.

Indeed, our expectations for our own old age should be tempered by the fact that how we age is subject to considerable variation. The biggest single correlation with the number of years post-retirement spent in good health is education: people who have degrees live both longer and healthier lives than those who do not.[6] Depending on how you look at it, education feeds into affluence, or affluence feeds into education, but the result is that people from the least deprived areas live up to 15 years longer in good health than those from the most deprived.[7] Our expectations for retirement may, or may not, correlate with what we can reasonably expect, but in defining the normal aspiration, we fail to account for the fact that not everyone can expect the same.

Health in old age and wealth are inextricably linked: one needs sufficient wealth to have a reasonable expectation of a healthy old age, and one needs sufficient wealth to be able to afford a decent retirement. Camilla Cavendish argues that it would be fairer and more affordable to base retirement age on years left to live rather than time worked.[8] Given that affluence is broadly determined by the affluence of the family in which one grows up, one wonders if she has a point. Of course, there is individual variation, but across the whole population, the life prospects for children in more affluent families are markedly more positive.[9] This does not just raise questions about retirement ages for the most affluent – the different prognosis for old age according to income poses big questions for social policy.

A simple reality that is already facing us is the idea that our longer lives already mean that our current arrangements for retirement are unsustainable. This is the point made by Lynda Gratton and Andrew Scott in their book *The 100-Year Life*,[10] in which they highlight that the skills we enter the job market with will no longer sustain us for an entire career. Indeed, they argue that younger people are already planning for working lives comprising multiple different career strands, incorporating rest and reinvention in their own narrative arcs. Even though the scope for change is large, and people's plans have already altered, there is no scent of adaptation, for example, in our patterns of education. We still cohort people by age and track them up the educational elevator, dropping them off at different age-defined exit points. Higher education, for example, could adapt around this new reality to encourage educational opportunities to be taken at multiple and different life points.

It is not just longevity that will alter our working lives: demographic changes will reduce the available workforce: each year in the UK, 1.5 million people leave the workforce and only 750,000 enter;[11] and that is before we factor in the Brexit-driven repatriation of EU nationals who contributed so significantly to many and varied industries in the UK.

The reduction of people in work presents us with three choices: work longer, allow much greater levels of immigration or accept a lower quality of life. It is fanciful to predict that technology will bridge the labour gap. However good robots and AI become at elements of our productivity, both the rate of decline of the working-age population and the ongoing need for human skills means that we will spend the next 50 years running to keep up with the demand for workforce.

Yuval Harari[12] points out that the nature of work has already changed significantly. Technology changes the work we do, but it does not reduce the number of people required. The impact of automation in the workplace so far has been to hollow out the job market and replace middle-paying jobs. In their place, low-paid, insecure jobs with few non-pay benefits have been created. This has been a profound shift in our working lives, which raises fundamental questions about the value of labour. On another day, perhaps, I will outline the complex and profound challenge this presents to our social contract, but today, I will only emphasise that there have been significant alterations to the careers of the future when compared with the careers of the past. There is now a triple risk of less security, fewer benefits and lower pay, which renders redundant any plans for future old age based on present career assumptions.

There is therefore much to consider, but a laissez-faire approach will be insufficient: Daniel Kahneman[13] points out that we often resort to 'delusional optimism' when planning for the future. Such optimism should be punctured by learning that a man born in 1945 would have to save 4.5% of his salary to retire aged 65 on half his salary, while someone born in 1998 would have to save 25% to achieve the same.[14]

With the understanding that our working lives ought to last longer comes the possibility that our working lives could become more varied and interesting. Healthy ageing is associated with remaining active, connecting with people and retaining a sense of purpose.[15] Thus, the necessity of multistage working lives could become a positive change, cementing a lasting role for older people in the economy, wider society and their communities. However, the risk, and indeed the trajectory we are already on, is that we will instead find ourselves on a relentless treadmill of serial insecure and low-paid jobs. The nature of our later lives depends, therefore, on a collective decision about how we reward the labour of our workforce. The extent to which the government and social policy is willing and able to support the necessary ecosystem for a rapidly adaptable, appropriate remunerated workforce is a big question.

The inclusion of older people in a more lasting function in the productive economy hinges on our ability to incorporate changing capabilities as we age and modification to traditional career trajectories. More philosophically, however, it requires us to appreciate the state of intergenerational relationships in the present. The spectre of intergenerational conflict emerges at the interface of generalisation, both by the young of the old and vice versa. Loose characterisations are unhelpfully reductive – that older people all enjoy foreign holidays and gold-plated pensions and younger people squander their money on avocados instead of houses. It is unseemly and it is inaccurate – but there are important truths to consider.

The Economist[16] highlights that it is millennials who lost the most from the 2008 financial crash and it is young people now who stand to lose the most from the coronavirus pandemic. However, a counterpoint is important: Age UK[17] estimates that 2.1 million pensioners (18%) live below the poverty line. Furthermore, 5 million grandparents (40%) provide regular care for their grandchildren, with the majority doing so every week.[18]

What this reveals is that intergenerational relationships are being altered right now in the structure and function of modern families, which in turn affects the opportunity to care for older people. Family structures in the last 50 years have been altered by shifting cultural norms and demographic changes; longevity and reduced fertility have created 'beanpole' families, in which multiple generations co-exist, with fewer young people than just two generations ago. Adults often have more grandparents than they have children. Further complication is added by the effects of divorce and remarriage, creating complex, extended and interwoven families.

These changes can have profound effects on how families relate to each other. In our daily lives, we are less members of Generation X, Y or Z than we are actors in an ever-changing social, demographic and economic landscape.

Durkheim[19] describes how the nature of family solidarity has become 'mechanical' rather than 'organic' in a faster changing society with new, multiple, interlacing and emerging rituals.[20] There exists, today, therefore, competition between different meanings, values and behaviours within multigenerational, multi-partnership families that are not captured well in the caricatures of modern discourse. At the very least, our plans for how we care for older people ought to reflect the prevalent normal variation in family structures. People do not arrive in old age unheralded and out of the context of their families, but current policy and practice too often pretends that they do.

Policies directed at specific age groups often tilt sympathies away from that group through the implied suggestion that they are special. The segregation in policy and practice of people by age pollutes our assumptions. There is a need for both age-agnostic approaches to life and policies that purposefully integrate people of all ages through defining people by roles and capabilities rather than years lived.

Family structures have changed seismically, but not in isolation. They have been accompanied, perhaps even driven, by important economic currents. Capitalism, from the 1970s onwards, has heralded greater instability of employment[21] in a shift to transient jobs with fewer benefits. Phillipson[22] describes an 'undertow of instability and crisis' in which incomes fluctuate, pension plans close and governments extend working life by moving the state retirement age further away. The emerging economy is a system of 'disorganised capitalism' where even traditionally affluent professional groups feel financially vulnerable. Transient job loss becomes normal and the risk of managing future pension and social care costs has become an almost purely private concern.

In this context, individuals necessarily become more selfish: the provision for a comfortable retirement requires the accumulation of wealth. If employers do not provide good pensions as a benefit, and the government is not interested in risk-pooling, the actions of individuals will necessarily adapt.

In this vein, we should contrast the universal provision of healthcare with the private provision of social care. In both health and social care, the costs are potentially huge and unequally distributed, but only in healthcare do we protect individuals from potentially catastrophic costs. In social care, the state only steps in when assets and savings have been spent. Those with the means and the knowledge take actions to protect their assets. As Kate Raworth describes in *Doughnut Economics*,[23] money changes behaviour. Contemporary policy around social care and retirement encourages individual action, which may come at the expense of a collective response in a way that is unfamiliar to those of us who work in the NHS.

In this way, the NHS has become less an emblem of our social attitudes and more a moral offset. It is a legacy of past aspirations whose preservation reflects well on us today. We do not enact services that demonstrate our willingness to pool risk as a society – a truth tellingly revealed by our collective failure to address the gross inequities of social care funding.

The rise of individual and private responsibility for unpredictable risks as we age (the need for expensive care is unpredictable and uninsurable) highlights the rising silhouette of inequality. Problems that express themselves in later life – such as years spent in ill-health, life expectancy, the ability to afford social care and pensioner poverty – find their roots much, much earlier in life. Thus, the nature of old age in the UK today is founded in the issues of fairness and its cousin, equality.

For example, at the outset of the coronavirus lockdown, it was noticeable how dependent we all were for our daily necessities on the lower-paid members of our society. The work of supermarket staff, refuse collectors and delivery drivers, as well as healthcare staff and the police, are part of our social commons: these workers do not themselves generate revenue for their employers, but they allow all of us to live better than we could without them. Too often these important jobs are paid poorly, so that the people who provide us with the basic elements of civilisation are themselves people too worried about meeting the costs of today to have the time to worry about meeting the costs of their future.

This is a crucial facet of understanding old age today: the nature of life in old age is influenced by health (which is a function of childhood affluence and education) and wealth; the nature of pensions is dependent on the nature of employment; the affordability of social care is a function of accumulated wealth or the good fortune not to need much. Thus, quality of life in old age is as much a function of economics as social or healthcare factors.

At a time when employment has become more precarious and benefits less generous, we have learned through the pandemic that the people society relies on are our lowest-paid neighbours. Yet alongside such changes to the nature of employment, public services have been eroded. The austerity programme from 2010 reduced social benefits and disproportionately affected the poorest and youngest neighbourhoods. In the UK, a majority of poor households have at least one person in work, meaning that work no longer pays. This is the context in which we have to think about a society increasingly comprised of older people.

Within this framework comes the appreciation of the corrosive quality of inequality. The Equality Trust shows that since 1979 inequality has increased, peaking in 1990 and remaining flat ever since.[24] Inequality itself has a toxic effect on society. Richard Wilkinson and Kate Pickett[25] illustrate that overall societal welfare flows from higher equality than it does from national wealth. More equal societies are happier and healthier, even when they are poorer. Furthermore, high levels of inequality equate to higher rates of environmental degradation: the pursuit of wealth trumps the protection of the natural resources and the environment.

The NHS, for example, is not special because of the care it delivers but because of the solidarity that binds it together. We could decide that the same solidarity could underpin both social care and our wider welfare state, and it could have a meaningful benefit to the lives of most people, not least older people.

A wider perspective is useful to appreciate the breadth of issues that feed into the nature of old age in the UK today and the range of actions required to make real the prospect of a fulfilling old age. It is also a mirror to the reality that for the last decade, the health service has been poorly treated by a government representing a society that has probably undervalued the NHS for some time. The risk we run is that by winding, or grinding, the health service into the ground, we will lose sight of the one service that illustrates the potential for collective, societal responses to problems that land unpredictably and catastrophically. I suspect that if it goes, it will be gone forever, and much of the potential to create a positive context for ageing in the UK will disappear with it.

I cannot, with sufficient brevity, begin to outline the solutions required. Instead, my point is to illustrate that it is insufficient to view the aetiology of problems in old age as challenges only for health and social care services. It is an oft-quoted maxim that the measure of a society is how it treats its weakest members, but my point is broader – there is something equally telling in how well a society protects its members from enfeeblement in the first place.

Endnotes

1   Hagestad, G. O. and Uhlenberg, P. (2005) 'The social separation of old and young: A root of ageism.' *Journal of Social Issues 1*, 2, 343–360.

2   Kohli, M. (1986) 'The World We Forgot: An Historical Review of the Life Course.' In V. W. Marshall (ed.), *Later Life*. Beverly Hills, CA: Sage Publications.

3   Diamond, J. (2012) *The World Until Yesterday*. London: Penguin Books.

4   Pasupathi, M. and Lochenhoff, C. E. (2002) 'Ageist Behaviour.' In T. D. Nelson (ed.), *Ageism: Stereotyping and Prejudice Against Older Persons*. Cambridge, MA: MIT Press.

5   Hagestad and Uhlenberg (2005), p.351.

6   Cavendish, C. (2019) *Extra Time*. London: Harper Collins.

7   *Ibid.*

8   *Ibid.*

9   Social Mobility Commission (2019) *Class Privilege Remains Entrenched as Social Mobility Stagnates*. Accessed on 18/2/2022 at www.gov.uk/government/news/class-privilege-remains-entrenched-as-social-mobility-stagnates.

10 Gratton, L. and Scott, A. (2017) *The 100-Year Life*. London: Bloomsbury.

11 Cavendish (2019).

12 Harari, Y. (2016) *Homo Deus: A Brief History of Tomorrow*. London: Vintage Press.

13 Kahneman, D. (2012) *Thinking, Fast and Slow*. London: Penguin, p.252.

14 Gratton and Scott (2017).

15 Cavendish (2019).

16 The Economist (2020) 'Unlucky millennials.' *The Economist*, April 16, 2020.

17 Age UK (2021) *Poverty in Later Life*. Accessed on 18/2/2022 at www.ageuk.
    org.uk/globalassets/age-uk/documents/policy-positions/money-matters/
    poverty_in_later_life_briefing_june_2021.pdf.

18 Age UK (2017) *5 Million Grandparents Take On Childcare Responsibilities*. Accessed
    on 18/2/2022 at www.ageuk.org.uk/latest-news/articles/2017/september/
    five-million-grandparents-take-on-childcare-responsibilities.

19 Durkheim, E. (1933) *The Division of Labour in Society*. New York: Free Press.

20 Katz, R. and Lowenstein, A. (2010) 'Theoretical Perspectives on Intergenerational
    Solidarity, Conflict and Ambivalence.' In M. Izuhara (ed.), *Ageing and Intergen-
    erational Relations: Family Reciprocity from a Global Perspective*. Bristol: Policy
    Press.

21 Lash, S. and Urry, J. (1987) *The End of Organised Capitalism*. Cambridge: Polity
    Press.

22 Phillipson, C. (2010) 'Globalisation, global ageing and intergenerational change.'
    In M. Izuhara (ed.), *Ageing and Intergenerational Relations: Family Reciprocity from
    a Global Perspective*. Bristol: Policy Press, p.20.

23 Raworth, K. (2017) *Doughnut Economics: Seven Ways to Think like a 21st Century
    Economist*. London: Random House.

24 The Equality Trust (n.d.) *How Has Inequality Changed?* Accessed on 18/2/2022
    at https://equalitytrust.org.uk/how-has-inequality-changed.

25 Wilkinson, R. G. and Pickett, K. (2010) *The Spirit Level: Why Greater Equality
    Makes Society Stronger*. London: Bloomsbury Press.

Maurice and Stanley

Maurice grew up in Henley, attended grammar school and left Oxford in 1949 with a third-class degree in Classics. A little time later, he started work for a multinational company. He speaks little about the nature of his work, except to remark that he was posted for periods to West Africa, the Middle East and the Far East. His easy manner of conversation, even now in his mid-90s, reveals his talent for benign chat. He is certainly very good at it. He tells stories with a great sense of setting and embellishes them with the little details that bring them to life. It is a skill he seems to have honed over many years and even perhaps used professionally.

His career lasted 30 years and he retired in his late 50s on a generous final salary pension, which he still draws today. With the lump sum pension payments plus some savings, he bought a piece of land in Mid Dorset and built a house. It is not to my taste, with its alpine aspect of a broad, external chimney breast and steeply sloping roof. While supervising the construction of the house, he fell in love with Dorset and moved down full-time with his wife when building was complete. The house is large and the gardens extensive, with wonderful views across the valley beyond, where sheep graze, buzzards hover and the rhythms of rural life echo around.

His children and later his grandchildren and great-grandchildren often stay and so numerous are they that there is usually someone visiting.

His is a comfortable and enjoyable existence, yet if it weren't for the house, it would be difficult to guess what his impact on the world has been. His career was never a passion for him, only ever the means to a comfortable, unharried existence, followed by a comfortable, unharried retirement.

At the time I met him, he had been drawing the pension he paid into for 30 years for over 40.

The effortlessness of Maurice's life contrasts with Stanley's. Stanley grew up in a poor and large family in Fortuneswell, Portland. Fortuneswell hugs the steep slopes that connect the lower reaches of the islands to the quarrying community up above. It is achingly poor, even today. The rivalry between those at the top of the island and those at the bottom has a ferocity that is only possible between near neighbours.

As Portlanders, Stanley's family was intimately connected to the sea and scratched a living fishing. It was no surprise, then, when at the outbreak of the Second World War, Stanley enlisted in the Royal Navy. He spent much of the war on a battleship, deployed to the Arctic and later to the Pacific. Stanley was present when Rear Admiral Harcourt accepted the Japanese surrender in Hong Kong.

After the war, Stanley returned to Portland and moved into a house near his family. He still lives in this house today. Initially, he worked as a fisherman, before training as an electrician and then working for the council. He married a local girl and they raised three children together. Two of them still live in Portland, while the third is across the ferry bridge in Weymouth.

Stanley retired from the council when he was 65 and continues to live in his little house with his wife. With his modest company pension and the state pension, he lives comfortably enough, but he cannot afford any more ambitious plans. His house still does not have central heating, and they continue to use a coal-fired Rayburn for their cooking and heating. There is a toilet upstairs and one outside, but there is not one downstairs.

Stanley's knees give him trouble, which makes the stairs a bit of a nuisance. In recent years, he has converted the spare bedroom into a lounge, and he stays upstairs most days, watching the racing on the large, flat-screen television his son installed for him. It's colder upstairs, away from the Rayburn, but at least he doesn't have to do the stairs.

CHAPTER 14

So What?

When I started writing this book, my goal was to share with you what I know about living in old age and dying. I wanted to illuminate through stories and analysis what my medical practice has taught me. What has emerged is something slightly different. The process of writing has asked me to trace back the problems I outline to their origins, and it has been an education for me to pull the strands and observe just how far back they extend.

To me, Chapter 1 feels a long way away and a long time ago. I wonder, half-jokingly, if I am different now, but by lifting our gaze, we have scanned the wider horizons that channel us to this final moment. I hope that you have found it instructive.

Yet, we still need to address the problem of 'so what?' What use is insight into the advantages and challenges of the present unless it informs our actions in the future? An appreciation for the modern context of dying, ageing and living helps us paint the ideal form of the future.

The appropriation of death by medicine has rendered us unfamiliar with it, leaving us too often unprepared for the death of loved ones, as well as our own. Discourse about medicine pitches us in battle with disease and mortality, but it is a fight that we are doomed to lose, always. It is a fight that creates an illusion of our individual influence: if someone survives cancer because they fought it, does someone die from it because they didn't?

Thus, when considering the medical care of older people and those with frailty, the answer to the question, 'What does success look like?' is necessarily characterised by your own frame of reference to medicine, ageing and dying. Mine is altered by my daily familiarity with the sights, sounds and smells of ageing, and my own personal demon is to fight the spectre of clinical nihilism. As we consider in general terms what it means to be mortal, and what the role for medicine is as we age, we would do well to reconcile ourselves to unalterable realities and pause to consider our own personal meanings. What we need from health and social care services should be informed by what we can realistically hope for in old age and shaped accordingly.

Taking one step back from mortality takes us to the experience of living in old age today and the understanding that old age, as experienced today, is a modern phenomenon – in which we are amateurs. Ageing may be further delayed through better understanding and management of the lifestyle factors that drive senescence, but immortality requires both a medical technology that does not exist (and may not be technically possible) and careful consideration of the ethics and philosophy of eternal life. Ageing is not just a biological problem, it is a central part of what it means to be alive, to be human. The ambition for empiricism in medicine does not itself justify a subjugation of life in its entirety to that same empiricism. Life remains, at least in part, a function of meaning and morality.

Importantly, individual perspective about life and the world changes with age – based on experience for which there is no shortcut. Life must be lived. The relative absence of our elders' perspectives in the world impoverishes us all and amplifies our general myopia about mortality; it contributes to our neglect of the nature of life for older people. This problem exists in microcosm in medical practice, where the reactive nature of practice, allied to the tendency towards curative intent, ignores the importance of the dying role and helps sustain the widespread hope that perhaps each of us will be the first human to not die.

Thus, the role for doctors in ageing and dying should be more circumscribed than it currently is. There is a clear function for doctors in the treatment of long-term conditions, the diagnosis of new ones and the articulation of treatment options. However, a misplaced confidence in current levels of medical knowledge is revealed by the question, 'How much time do I have left?' It is a question that can only ever be answered with a wide margin of error.

In fact, it is not time left that matters as much as the ability and space to attend to spiritual needs (i.e. the search for meaning), yet it is this crucial aspect of the dying role that is exorcised too often from the dying process through the medicalisation of ageing and dying. This has occurred in an increasingly secular world, abandoning not just the belief system of religion, but also the established rituals that enable both individuals and communities to cope with death through the formalised habits and learning of our forebears.

We seem to be in the process of recasting ourselves as a technological species, but the issue of ageing and dying is not only a technological challenge. The characterisation of ageing and dying as a collection of medical problems, as well as the casting of frailty as a long-term medical problem, is not false, but it is oversimplified. A medical view of old age is a narrow view of old age. Good healthcare is only one element of good care for older people, and it doesn't begin to address important aspects of ageing that contribute to poor health, such as social isolation and loneliness.

Raising the spotlight from the nature of health services for older people shines a light on both their role in society generally and the isolation of the NHS as a public service truly designed for public good. It is a reminder that the NHS, as a comprehensive healthcare service, free at the point of use, based on need and not ability to pay, represents a historic value set not currently in vogue today. When one looks at how public services outside the NHS support older people, particularly social care, there is a glaring absence of an NHS-like ethos.

Not only does this reveal that in an increasingly ageing society, more demands are being placed on ever more pressured health and social care structures, it also illuminates our collective tendency to plan for old age by hoping that we will individually be OK. Optimism is not a strategy.

As I've shown, healthcare services can adapt easily enough around the needs of older people if one accepts healthcare as only one aspect of good care and appreciates the room for personal subjectivity in defining what success looks like. However, the delegation of care of older people to poorly treated health and social care staff exposes either a poor appreciation of the value of the work they do or ignorance of the general level of need; and just as demand has increased, health and social care have been weakened by the impact of austerity over ten years. Does this neglect of important public services tell us something about the leadership of our public services and government, or does our collective tolerance of it reveal something more generally damning?

There is certainly the sense that we value neoliberal economic thinking over the nurture of non-economic motivations and benefits. In particular, we forget that many people, not least the staff of the NHS, are genuinely motivated by the opportunity to do their jobs well and care for patients to a high standard. The capacity for ambition, altruism and goodness exists outside purely financial considerations. Yet current practices for performance management not only discount intrinsic motivation for good work, but in fact stifle it entirely by denying its existence.

Better healthcare services are possible and necessary, but it is more than just a question of money: we must pay attention to the conditions and resources with which the work is done, invest in teams and individuals and appreciate that healthcare staff are people too, not just units of activity. Witness how recent events have contributed to moral injury, staff burnout and resignation to understand that concern for staff is only optional if you don't care about the quality of healthcare.

The more time I have spent reflecting on the nature of services required to serve our older people well, the more I have realised that the adaptation of health and social care can only address some of the need. Indeed, the mounting pressure being placed on health and social care services in the management of ageing is not only a function of demographics: it is problem exacerbated by wider social issues, such as age segregation.

The habit of age segregation colours the lives of our oldest neighbours, who too often find themselves in advanced frailty cut off from the routines of the rest of society. The toxic effects of social isolation can be seen in the health effects of loneliness, but there is also a bigger story to be told: the absence of older people from routine social interaction denies wider society the benefit of having them around – from improved relationships and appreciation between different age groups to better team functioning and productivity in the workplace and a better understanding of the realities of ageing.

Age segregation is just one example, but it is one founded on the age-agnostic problems of inequality and insecurity, which themselves are disguised through the blurring discourse about intergenerational conflict. In present times, it is younger people who have suffered the greatest loss from the pandemic and the Great Recession. This could be presented as intergenerational unfairness, as it often is. However, this is an oversimplification. In the context of rapid demographic changes, people are already living, and adapting to, the realities of altered demographics. Family structures have changed but cannot be said to have broken down. Look at the prevalence of grandparent support in childcare and the need for parental support in house purchases for first-time buyers.

While this may take us away from the message about the core needs of older people, it is a key point: there is no point adapting around the needs of older people now if the needs of the older people of the future will be different as a result of social, economic and demographic trends visible right now. Bobby Duffy[1] distinguishes between period effects, lifecycle effects and cohort effects, observing that if we rely on when someone was born to explain their attitudes, beliefs and experiences, we are relying too much on cohort effects. Much of the difference in experience between younger and older people at the same stages of life needs to be understood in terms of how our lifecycles have altered and how the period of time we exist in now has changed our expectations and reality.

The changes we are currently experiencing are significant, and will undoubtedly feed into differences in the nature and length of our working lives, which will inevitably feed into differences in the nature of our old age. Assumptions about professional careers and the nature of employment have altered markedly in a short space of time. Each of these changes is the germ of change in expectations for old age and we will be able to track the effects over the years.

Consider, for example, how the job market has been altered by the hollowing out of middle-skilled jobs, creating more dependence on insecure, poorly paid work with few non-pay benefits. This change by itself heralds a future of less secure and later retirement than we have become accustomed to over the last 50 years.

It is not the only change: job security has waned in a world in which wealth inequality is rising, while at the same time we are adjusting to the emerging realities of pandemic diseases, environmental degradation and global heating. These changes give further context to the question, 'What matters most?', and I cannot shake the suspicion that while it remains a question that will forever be valid to ask of those in the final phase of their life, it is also a question we ought to start asking of ourselves more generally. It raises fundamental questions about how we prioritise a whole range of issues, including education, social care and welfare.

If we use the mirror of old age to understand the flaws in our society, we learn that the quality of life in old age is currently built on luck: the good fortune to remain healthy and cognitively intact and the good fortune to have material wealth. None of this is individually earned, and the ill-health, poverty or social isolation of older people will never be addressed without collective action. It is too great a task for us all to tackle it individually.

Instead comes the recognition that improving old age is founded on improving life for all ages and that the time is right for a review of our implicit social contract. In a world where, increasingly, work doesn't pay subsistence costs, where wealth is unequal and where current lifestyles are causing the existential threats of pandemic illness and climate change, we need to review our guiding value set.

It is my contention that the lives of our elders today, and in the future, are constrained by the political, economic and social choices we have made in the last 30 years and that improving the lives of older people in particular will flow inevitably from addressing the inequalities and insecurities felt by all age groups at present. Fixing the problems of a specific group of people does not necessitate a bespoke response but instead requires the addressing of the visible generic issues.

The quality of the lives of older people cannot be measured only in financial terms. Social inclusion and meaning are important for all of us, not just older people, but it is the limitations of frailty and old age that raise their absence to our awareness. Thus, as we deepen our appreciation of the nature of ageing and dying in the UK today and understand better the systems needed to service the needs of an ageing population, those threads we have pulled on reveal themselves to be both long and extensively intertwined.

Remember that story about Graham and his reaction to the baby I took with me on my ward round? That captures the importance of hope in our lives and the ambition to create a world that cycles on contentedly after we have gone. It is that hope and that ambition that should drive us as we look to a future with enormous challenges. It is that hope and that ambition that will sustain us and reward us. It is that hope and ambition that is missing from our lives today. Let us find it and restore it.

Endnotes

1   Duffy, B. (2021) *Generations: Does When You're Born Shape Who You Are?* London: Atlantic Books.